ABC of
Patient Safety

ABC series

The revised and updated ABC series – written by specialists for non-specialists

- With over 40 titles, this extensive series provides a quick and dependable reference on a broad range of topics in all the major specialities

- An easy-to-use resource, covering the symptoms, investigations, treatment and management of conditions presenting in your day-to-day practice

- Full colour photographs and illustrations aid diagnosis and patient understanding of a condition

- Each book in the new series now offers links to further information and articles, and a new dedicated website provides even more support

- A highly illustrated, informative and practical source of knowledge for GPs, GP registrars, junior doctors, doctors in training and those in primary care

For further information on the entire ABC series, please visit:

www.abcbookseries.com

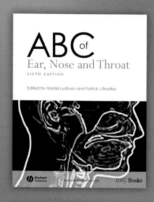

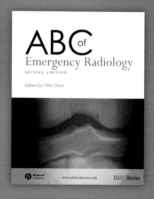

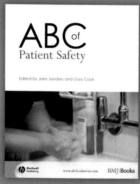

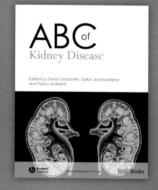

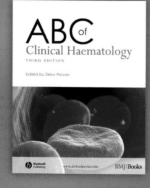

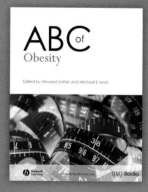

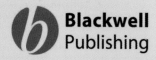
Blackwell Publishing

BMJ|Books

ABC of
Patient Safety

EDITED BY

John Sandars
Senior Lecturer in Community Based Education
Medical Academic Education Unit, University of Leeds, Leeds, UK

Gary Cook
Consultant Epidemiologist, Stepping Hill Hospital
Stockport NHS Foundation Trust, Stockport, UK
Honorary Senior Fellow in Public Health
University of Manchester, Manchester, UK

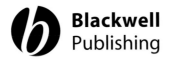
Blackwell Publishing

BMJ|Books

Blackwell Publishing, Inc., 350 Main Street, Malden, Massachusetts 02148-5020, USA
Blackwell Publishing Ltd, 9600 Garsington Road, Oxford OX4 2DQ, UK
Blackwell Publishing Asia Pty Ltd, 550 Swanston Street, Carlton, Victoria 3053, Australia

First published 2007

1 2007

Library of Congress Cataloging-in-Publication Data
ABC of patient safety / edited by John Sandars and Gary Cook.
     p. ; cm.
 Includes bibliographical references.
 ISBN 978-1-4051-5692-9
 1. Hospital care--Safety measures. 2. Hospital care--Quality control. I. Sandars, John,
MB. II. Cook, Gary, 1952-
 [DNLM: 1. Patient Care--standards. 2. Medical Errors--prevention & control. 3. Safety
Management--methods. W 84.1 A134 2007]

 RA972.A234 2007
 362.11028'9--dc22

                                                         2006035609
ISBN: 978-1-4051-5692-9

A catalogue record for this title is available from the British Library

Cover image of handwashing by a member of hospital staff is courtesy of John Cole/
Science Photo Library

Set in Minion 9.25/12pt by Sparks, Oxford – www.sparks.co.uk
Printed and bound in Singapore by Fabulous Printers Pte Ltd

Associate Editor: Vicki Donald
Editorial Assistant: Victoria Pittman
Production Controller: Rachel Edwards

For further information on Blackwell Publishing, visit our website:
www.blackwellpublishing.com

Contents

Contributors

Darren M Ashcroft

Clinical Senior Lecturer, School of Pharmacy and Pharmaceutical Sciences, University of Manchester, Manchester, UK

Maureen Baker

Special Clinical Adviser, National Patient Safety Agency, London, UK

Martin Beyer

Senior Researcher in Quality Improvement and Patient Safety, Institute for General Practice, Frankfurt, Germany

Judith A Cantrill

Professor of Medicines (Usage, Evaluation and Policy), School of Pharmacy and Pharmaceutical Sciences, University of Manchester, Manchester, UK

Tanya Claridge

Professional Development Advisor and Health Visitor, Stockport Primary Care Trust, Stockport, UK

Jenny Firth-Cozens

Special Adviser on Modernisation of Postgraduate Education, London Deanery, London, UK

Keith Haynes

Director, MPS Risk Consulting Ltd, Leeds, UK

Amanda Howe

Professor of Primary Care, School of Medicine, Health Policy and Practice, University of East Anglia, Norwich, UK

Michael Jones

Professor of Common Law, University of Liverpool, Liverpool, UK

Peter J Nicklin

Associate Consultant with the Medical Protection Society and Honorary Senior Lecturer at the University of Leeds Medical School, UK

Robert L Phillips

Director of the Robert Graham Centre for Policy Studies in Family Medicine and Primary Care, The Robert Graham Centre, Washington DC, USA

Julie Price

Clinical Risk Manager, MPS Risk Consulting Ltd, Leeds, UK

Julie Rohe

Research Scientist, Agency for Quality in Medicine, Berlin, Germany

Aziz Sheikh

Professor of Primary Care Research and Development, Division of Community Health Sciences, University of Edinburgh, UK

Richard Thomson

Director of Epidemiology and Research, National Patient Safety Agency, London, UK; Professor of Epidemiology and Public Health, Institute of Health Sciences, Newcastle University, Newcastle upon Tyne, UK

Peter Walsh

Chief Executive, Action Against Medical Accidents, Croydon, UK

Preface

It is a sad fact that healthcare can actually harm the people that it should be helping. This is true and alarming. However, healthcare is a complex process, and it is not surprising that patient safety can be threatened.

Our aim in writing this book has been to offer a practical approach to understanding and improving patient safety in both primary and secondary care. We fully accept that we have only provided a small snapshot into the ever-expanding world of patient safety.

However, we believe that if the basic principles were applied then patient safety would substantially improve.

We would like to thank all of the contributors for their hard work in bringing together the large amount of existing knowledge, the National Patient Safety Agency (NPSA) for reviewing the manuscript to ensure that it fits into current trends, and the editorial team at Blackwell Publishing.

John Sandars
Gary Cook

CHAPTER 1

The Scope of the Problem

John Sandars

OVERVIEW

- Many patients are harmed by healthcare, both secondary and primary, and often this harm is preventable
- The frequency and nature of threats to patient safety depend on the method of identification and classification
- Adverse drug events are the commonest threat to patient safety in secondary care
- Failure and delay in diagnosis is the commonest threat to patient safety in primary care

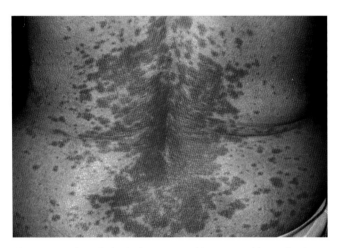

Figure 1.1 Rash on the back of an 80-year-old man caused by an allergic reaction to the antifungal drug terbinafine. (Reproduced by courtesy of Dr P. Marazzi, Science Photo Library.)

Patient safety is a major concern for all healthcare providers. It appears perverse that patients can suffer harm when they are being treated and cared for. However, healthcare is complex and its outcome is influenced by many factors. It is inevitable that within any healthcare system patients will be harmed, and in every encounter there is the potential for harm to occur. This has been recognized since the time of the physicians of Ancient Greece and Rome – 'First, do no harm.'

How frequent are threats to patient safety?

In the 1970s, research identified that as many as 36% of admissions to a general medical unit and 13% of admissions to intensive care units followed adverse events in which patients had been harmed, most often as a result of medications (Fig. 1.1). However, it was the publication of the Harvard Medical Practice Study (HMPS) in 1991 that highlighted to healthcare providers and policy-makers the extent of harm. Patient safety was now in the public eye, not only in the USA but throughout the world.

The HMPS analysed more than 30 000 randomly selected medical records of recently discharged patients from a random selection of 51 hospitals in New York State. Adverse events, defined as extended hospitalization, disability at the time of discharge, or death resulting from medical care, were identified. The proportion of hospital admissions experiencing an adverse event was 3.7%. The proportion of adverse events that were preventable was 58%. These findings were confirmed in a similar study of acute care hospitals in Colorado and Utah, with 2.9% of admissions experiencing an adverse event, of which 53% were preventable. The Quality in Aus-

tralian Health Care Study also analysed medical records, and found that 16.6% of hospital admissions experienced an adverse event (Table 1.1). Extrapolation of the results of both US studies implies that in 1997 between 44 000 and 98 000 US citizens died in hospital as a result of preventable adverse events. If these rates are typical of secondary care in the UK, then at least 850 000 admissions will experience an adverse event.

No similar research using systematic review of medical records has been performed in primary care. However, studies have used incident reporting in an attempt to estimate adverse events in primary care. One of the largest studies was performed in Australia, with 805 incidents from 324 general practitioners being analysed. The esti-

Table 1.1 US and Australian research into adverse events in hospitals

	Harvard Medical Practice Study, 1991	Quality in Australian Health Care Study, 1995
Proportion of inpatient episodes leading to harmful adverse events	3.7%	16.6%
Proportion of inpatient episodes resulting in permanent disability or death	0.7%	3%

mated rate of adverse events was 40–80 per 100 000 consultations, of which 76% were considered preventable and 27% had the potential for severe harm. In a study of prescriptions that had been issued by general practitioners in the UK and then reviewed by community pharmacists, a potential adverse drug reaction was identified in 0.13% of all prescriptions. These rates may initially appear to be insignificant, but it is important to consider that in the UK there are over one million general practitioner consultations each day, and 1.5 million prescriptions are generated daily.

What are the types of threat to patient safety?

Adverse drug events, defined as injuries resulting from medical intervention related to a drug, are the commonest threat to patient safety in secondary care. However, not all adverse drug events are preventable, such as an unexpected allergic reaction. In a review of 4031 adult admissions to 11 medical and surgical units at two hospitals in the USA, there was an event rate of 6.5 adverse drug events per 100 admissions, of which 28% were judged preventable. Adverse drug events are also common in primary care, with 13–51% of all reported adverse incidents related to medication. In two recent UK-based studies of admissions to hospital, about 6% were regarded as being the result of a preventable adverse drug event (Fig. 1.2).

In hospitals, other common types of adverse event are preventable infections, surgical and diagnostic mistakes, and events involving medical equipment (Fig. 1.3).

The medico-legal database of the Medical Protection Society (MPS) provides a useful source of information concerning 1000 consecutive formally registered claims that had been made against general practitioners in the UK, and is highly relevant to primary care. The largest category was Investigation and Treatment (63%), followed by Prescribing (19%). In the Investigation and Treatment category, the main types were failure or delay in diagnosis and referral to secondary care. The largest group was related to malignancy, followed by diseases of the circulatory system and injuries. In Prescribing, the main types were failure to warn or recognize drug side effects, followed by medi-

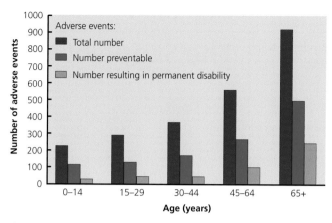

Figure 1.3 Numbers of adverse events, preventable adverse events, and events resulting in permanent disability, by age. (Adapted from Wilson RM *et al.*, 1995.)

cation error. This is an error at any stage of the medication process, including prescribing, dispensing, administering and monitoring. The main groups were related to the use of steroids in disease management and allergic reactions when antibiotics were prescribed. Administration problems were noted in 4.8% of claims, the main types being poor records, communication difficulties between members of the practice, and errors made by receptionists or other employees of the practice. Practice nurses were noted in 3.2% of claims, with the main types related to performing an injection or blood test, undertaking a procedure, and inappropriate advice.

Perspectives from patients and healthcare professionals

In a telephone survey of 1513 adults in the USA, 42% reported that they or a family member had experienced harm as a consequence of interacting with the healthcare system. This is supported by other studies. One-third of US physicians reported harm to themselves or their family as a consequence of healthcare, and in another study 16% of patients had experienced a medication error.

What is the cost of threats to patient safety?

In the USA, preventable adverse events have been estimated to cost $17–29 billion a year. This includes litigation costs and the resultant increased healthcare costs. The total economic impact, including lost income and disability, has been estimated to be $38–50 billion a year. In the UK, adverse events in hospitalized patients have been estimated to cost at least £2 billion each year for the additional days required in hospital.

In addition to these economic costs there are other consequences. The aftermath of an adverse event in which a patient has been harmed will have an impact on the psychological and social well-being of all who are involved in the incident, whether patient, family or healthcare professional. There are also wider aspects, with loss in public trust in the healthcare system.

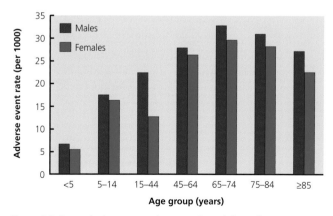

Figure 1.2 Rates of adverse events by age and sex. (After Aylin P, Tanna S, Bottle A, Jarman B. How often are adverse events reported in English hospital statistics? *Br Med J* 2004;**329**:369.)

Differences between studies

It is immediately apparent that there are wide differences between the various studies, and this is not only between secondary and primary care. When comparing studies it is important to consider the following points.

- **Purpose of data collection.** Studies have been performed for a variety of purposes. Some studies have had the main aim of identifying the frequency and nature of adverse events, but some have reviewed administrative and medico-legal databases. Such databases are more likely to include complaints that are unproven, contain details about more serious events, and not include events that have the potential to cause harm.
- **Settings.** There has been little extensive work from the UK, and most studies have been performed in the USA and Australia. These countries have differing approaches to healthcare, and comparison between countries with different healthcare systems may be inappropriate.
- **Definitions.** The definition of an 'adverse event' will determine what is identified, and what constitutes an adverse event varies considerably across various studies. Some studies have used a wider definition that encompassed actual and potential harm to patients whereas others considered only those that caused actual harm, including those resulting in medico-legal action. The classification of harm has often been made by a variety of people, ranging from individual doctors to administrative staff.
- **Method of data collection.** The identification of the true frequency requires a systematic process, similar to a mass screening programme for disease identification. Surveys have tried to capture the frequency in a hospital population, often by targeting specific groups, such as those receiving medication. However, such surveys are highly resource dependent, and opportunistic programmes have been more widely introduced, including primary care. Incident reporting, a type of opportunistic screening, does not give a true population frequency because it is limited to only those incidents that are reported. Most studies have been opportunistic, relying on the identification of incidents by self-reporting.
- **Classification.** The depth of understanding of threats to patient safety varies across the studies. Most studies have used simple classifications, such as prescribing, but this may oversimplify the cause.

It is easy to argue about the absolute frequency, types and cost of threats to patient safety, but the main message still stands: many patients are harmed by healthcare, both secondary and primary, and that harm is often preventable.

Further reading

Baker GR, Norton PG, Flintoft V *et al.* The Canadian Adverse Events Study: the incidence of adverse events among hospital patients in Canada. *Can Med Assoc J* 2004;**170**:1678–1686.

Brennan TA, Leape LL, Laird NM *et al.* Incidence of adverse events and negligence in hospitalized patients. Results of the Harvard Medical Practice Study I. *N Engl J Med* 1991;**324**:370–376.

Davis P, Lay-Yee R, Briant R *et al.* Adverse events in New Zealand public hospitals I: occurrence and impact. *New Zeal Med J* 2002;**115**:U271.

Davis P, Lay-Yee R, Briant R *et al.* Adverse events in New Zealand public hospitals II: preventability and clinical context. *New Zeal Med J* 2003;**116**:U624.

Department of Health Expert Group. *An Organisation with a Memory.* Department of Health, London, 2000.

Gawande AA, Thomas EJ, Zinner MJ, Brennan TA. The incidence and nature of surgical adverse events in Colorado and Utah in 1992. *Surgery* 1999;**126**:66–75.

Haynes K, Thomas M (eds) *Clinical Risk Management in Primary Care.* Radcliffe Medical Press, Oxford, 2005.

Leape LL, Brennan TA, Laird N *et al.* The nature of adverse events in hospitalized patients. Results of the Harvard Medical Practice Study II. *N Engl J Med* 1991;**324**:377–384.

Sandars J, Esmail A. *Threats to Patient Safety in Primary Care: A Review of the Research into the Frequency and Nature of Error in Primary Care.* Department of Health, London, 2002 (www.pcpoh.bham.ac.uk/publichealth/psrp/pdf/sanders_esmail_threats.pdf).

Vincent C, Neale G, Woloshynowych M. Adverse events in British hospitals: preliminary retrospective record review. *Br Med J* 2001;**322**:517–519.

Weingart SN, Wilson RMcL, Gibberd RW, Harrison B. Epidemiology of medical error. *Br Med J* 2000;**320**:774–777.

Wilson RM, Runciman WB, Gibberd RW *et al.* The Quality in Australian Health Care Study. *Med J Australia* 1995;**163**:458–471.

Further resources

National Patient Safety Agency (NPSA). Publications and more information are available from their website www.npsa.nhs.uk.

National Patient Safety Foundation (NPSF). Publications and more information are available from their website www.npsf.org.

CHAPTER 2

The Nature of Error

Jenny Firth-Cozens, John Sandars

OVERVIEW

- Most threats to patient safety are the result of a complex combination of active and latent failures
- Active failures are usually due to human factors
- Latent failures are mainly caused by underlying organizational problems and predispose to active failures
- Latent failures are the root cause of most threats to patient safety

Healthcare is inevitably associated with an increased risk of threats to patient safety. The problems that are presented are often complex and not easily defined. The response by healthcare workers is also complex, with a wide variety of healthcare workers working to deal with the problem, each using different approaches to manage the situation.

Why do threats to patient safety occur?

The investigation of many threats to patient safety has shown that there are usually multiple causes and they tend to occur when there is an unfortunate combination of 'active failures' and 'latent failures' (Fig. 2.1).

Active failures are usually associated with human factors. Occasionally there can be a sudden and unexpected failure of equipment

but this is rare. These active failures contribute to most threats to patients. However, latent failures are 'errors waiting to occur' and are associated with the healthcare system. These latent failures are the root cause of most active failures.

Human factors

Healthcare workers are at the 'sharp end' – professional expertise is applied, the effects are immediately noticed and it is where any threats to patient safety are seen.

At the sharp end, 'active failures' occur. Healthcare workers have to make decisions and actions occur that contribute to unsafe patient care (i.e. errors of commission). They may also omit key steps in a clinical task (i.e. errors of omission). These 'failures' are more likely if the healthcare worker is dealing with complex events, high levels of uncertainty, time pressures and fatigue (Box 2.1).

Cognitive psychology has identified the main types of error due to human factors (Fig. 2.2):
- **Slips.** These commonly occur when there is a distraction during a routine task. Examples include being interrupted whilst

> Box 2.1 **Early signs of a doctor in difficulties**
>
> - **The disappearing act:** lateness; excessive sick leave; not answering bleeps
> - **Low work rate:** slowness at making decisions, writing letters, finishing procedures
> - **Ward/surgery rage:** bursts of temper; shouting matches; real or imagined slights
> - **Rigidity:** poor tolerance of ambiguity; inability to compromise; difficulty prioritizing
> - **Bypass syndrome:** colleagues, nurses or patients find ways to avoid seeking his or her opinion or help
> - **Career problems:** difficulty with exams; uncertainty about career choice; disillusionment with medicine
> - **Insight failure:** rejection of constructive criticism; defensiveness; counter-challenge
>
> (Adapted from Paice E. The role of education and training. In: Cox J, King J, Hutchinson A, McAvoy, P. (eds), *Understanding Doctors' Performance*. Radcliffe Publishing, Oxford, 2005.)

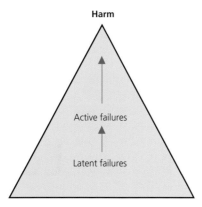

Figure 2.1 The pyramid of harm.

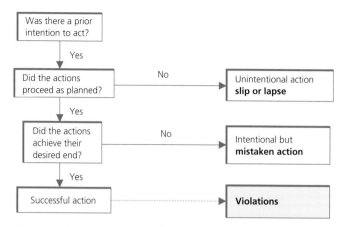

Figure 2.2 Intention–action algorithm. (Adapted from Reason, J. *Human Error*. Cambridge University Press, Cambridge, 1990.)

preparing an injection so that the wrong dose is drawn up into the syringe, and confusing the names of drugs when overtired. The person is not aware that the slip has occurred until after the event.
- **Lapses.** These occur when a standard approach, such as a protocol or guideline, is not followed. Individuals recognize that they are not following the particular advice but choose not to follow the advice. An example is when a healthcare worker is faced with a complex clinical situation and chooses not to follow a guideline because it does not easily apply to the problem that they are dealing with.
- **Mistakes.** These occur when there is a failure in judgement. Mistakes often occur when the healthcare professional has insufficient knowledge about a problem, either in diagnosis or in treatment. Alternatively, mistakes can also occur because an incorrect rule is applied to solve a problem – these types of errors are called rule-based mistakes.
- **Violation.** There is a deliberate attempt not to follow accepted approaches. These events are rare.

The healthcare system

Healthcare managers, policy-makers and regulators are at the 'blunt end' – they decide on how the care is delivered through policies, financial controls and management of the work of the healthcare professionals (Figs 2.3–2.4).

At the blunt end, 'latent conditions' occur (Box 2.2). A working environment is created that increases the probability that there will be an active failure at the sharp end. There are a lot of latent failures – all with the potential to cause an adverse event. An example is when the healthcare system is overloaded, such as overbooking admissions onto a ward. This may be compounded with insufficient staffing. Usually there is a combination of several small factors, each appearing to be insignificant when viewed alone (Box 2.3).

When latent failures occur in combination with only one active failure, such as a mistake in drug dose by a healthcare worker who is overtired because he or she has been working a series of long shifts, the result is a recipe for an adverse event to occur.

The role of the individual in patient safety

Until recently, the commonest approach to looking at patient safety has been to focus on the errors and violations of the individual healthcare worker. This has now changed to a systems approach, which sees causal factors as part of the system as a whole. However, the individual healthcare worker is a crucial factor in the provision of safe care, and it is important that this aspect is not ignored.

Recognizing individual problems

Some individual factors that impact on safety, such as inexperience or distractions, will apply to all healthcare workers at some point in their careers and so require organizational polices to address them. Other factors will be true for some individuals but not others, and these involve psychological or physical health problems, and par-

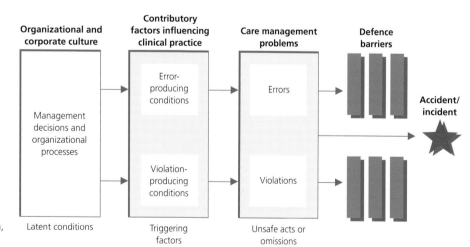

Figure 2.3 Stages of development of organizational accident. (Reproduced from Reason JT, Understanding adverse events: the human factor. In Vincent, CA, *Clinical Risk Management: Ensuring Patient Safety*, London, BMJ Books, 2001.)

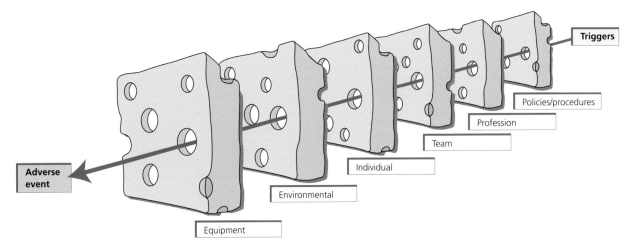

Figure 2.4 'Swiss cheese' diagram of error prevention. This model describes how a combination of several latent failures, each individually insufficient to cause an adverse event, can contribute to an adverse event. An active failure (the trigger) forms an adverse event by failing to be stopped by a series of barriers. The holes in these barriers act as latent failures in the system. (Adapted from Reason J. *Human Error*. Cambridge University Press, Cambridge, 1990.)

Box 2.2 **The main latent conditions for failure**

- Inadequate training
- Unworkable procedures
- Low standards of quality
- Poor or inadequate technology
- Unrealistic time pressures
- Understaffing

Box 2.3 **Factors in organizations where major catastrophes have occurred**

- Insufficient staffing and little or no slack
- Defective equipment
- An environment of poor information, uncertainty and stress
- Poor motivation and poor training

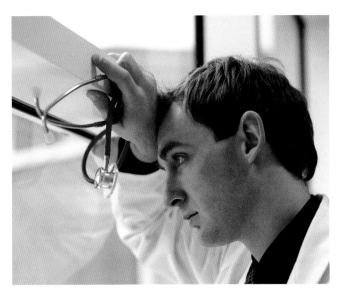

Figure 2.5 Stress and depression are particularly high in doctors. (Reproduced by courtesy of Mark Thomas/Science Photo Library.)

ticular personalities. Psychological problems include stress, depression, anxiety and psychotic disorders, as well as alcohol and other drug use (Fig. 2.5).

Stress and depression have been shown to be particularly high in doctors, and around 30% of doctors and other healthcare staff show above-threshold stress symptoms at any one time. In stress and depression, cognitive failures are frequent: concentration, memory and decision-making are reduced, and irritability often rises, making day-to-day work more difficult and interpersonal relationships strained. Healthcare organizations can have an indirect effect on the safety of patient care by providing an environment that keeps stress low: for example, by valuing staff, communicating well, providing clarity wherever they can, and reducing overload.

Psychiatric illnesses occur in doctors just as they do in the population as a whole. However, supervision, appraisal and revalidation procedures mean that risks are now regularly monitored. Doctors need to be open about mental health problems so that practice can stay safe, but this is less likely to happen in organizational cultures where disabled people are not valued or where team culture does not allow the open discussion of any difficulties that are posed.

Having a clear head

Alcohol use and abuse are also common among both male and female doctors and are often related to depression. Other drug abuse is also rising and is a major cause of referrals to programmes for impaired doctors in Australia. There remains a very tolerant culture within medicine that still tends to ignore its gravity and the consequences for the doctor and the patient.

Are some people naturally risky?

The concept of the risky personality has a long research literature, relating it primarily to increased activity in risky activities outside the workplace, but also shown to be related to less safe practices in healthcare workers. Risk perception also varies: some people can see danger more easily than others, with clear benefits to safety. This can be encouraged by increasing mental readiness. By visualizing each case (such as each operation) in advance it is possible to increase safety by anticipating the risks that might occur and how they might be remedied (Fig. 2.6).

Personality can play a part in unsafe care in other ways as well. Under stress the strengths and values of doctors can show a darker side: autonomy can become arrogance; competence can lead to a sense of invulnerability; the application of science may develop into being simply obstructive; and collegiality can become a conspiracy of silence.

Exhaustion

Risky behaviours are not just a function of personality, but can be increased through tiredness. Pilots subjected to strenuous night flights with sleep deprivation show increased impulsiveness as well as being clumsier and having lower mood. Increasing evidence from around the world shows that errors are more likely with overwork and a lack of sleep.

Technology and patient safety

The use of technology is ideal when large amounts of data have to be quickly managed. Computers do not get bored with repetitive tasks or become tired or stressed – the ideal conditions for humans to make errors.

Technology has a major role in the improvement of patient safety, as it does in all high-risk industries. Routine procedures can be replaced or monitored. Healthcare providers can be notified when there are deviations to the expected course, such as the use of an alarm to alert anaesthetists in an operating theatre when the patient's oxygen level falls. Decision-making can be improved, either at the time of diagnosis or when there are prescribing decisions (Fig. 2.7).

However, a paradox is that procedures that become highly reliant on technology can increase error because the operators still have human infallibility and may choose to ignore prompts or misinterpret information, especially if there is malfunction of the technology.

Patient safety can be improved by applying engineering principles to the design and evaluation of procedures. The use of technology usually requires a clear analysis of the task to be performed. This can identify potential problems and result in better-designed processes.

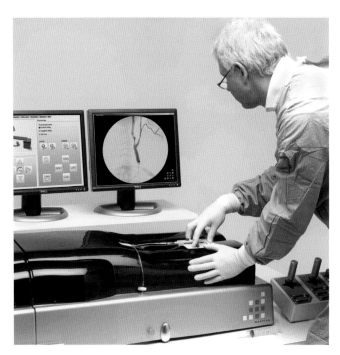

Figure 2.6 Simulation allows rehearsal of technical procedures. (Procedicus VIST™ – Vascular Intervention Simulation Trainer reproduced by courtesy of Mentice.)

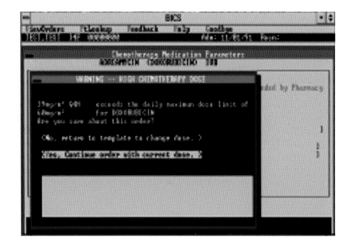

Figure 2.7 Computerized checking of a chemotherapy dose. (Reproduced from Bates DW, Using information technology to reduce rates of medication errors in hospital, *BMJ*, 2000; **320**:788–791.)

The importance of technology in the future development of patient safety will substantially increase. There will be increasing computerization of medical records and in the ordering and monitoring of prescribing. However, the greatest impact is likely to be the introduction of persuasive technologies that are designed to change people's attitudes and behaviours. Examples include devices that constantly monitor the performance of a surgeon and give feedback on performance, or those that help people to rehearse complex procedures.

Further reading

Nolan TW. System changes to improve patient safety. *Br Med J* 2000;**320**:771–773.

Reason J. Human error: models and management. *Br Med J* 2000;**320**:768–770.

Vincent C, Taylor-Adams S, Stanhope N. Framework for analysing risk and safety in clinical medicine. *Br Med J* 1998;**316**:1154–1157.

Further resources

BMA Counselling Service: provides doctors and their families with 24-hour telephone counselling by qualified counsellors. Tel. 0845 920 0169.

Sick Doctors' Trust, 36 Wick Crescent, Bristol BS4 4HG. Tel. helpline: 0870 4445163 (24 hrs). Website: www.sick-doctors-trust.co.uk

CHAPTER 3

Diagnosis

John Sandars

OVERVIEW

- Diagnosis is usually the first step in the process of healthcare, and errors in diagnosis are the commonest cause of threats to patient safety in primary and secondary care
- The results of diagnostic tests may be easily misinterpreted
- A common problem in the diagnostic process is doctor–patient communication, especially when there are different cultural aspects
- Poor management of results and referrals can lead to delayed diagnosis and patient harm

Diagnosis is the usual first step in any process of healthcare. Subsequent management is dependent on making an accurate diagnosis. Often a cascade of errors is set in place, with a sequence of errors in diagnosis and treatment that results in harm, or potential harm, to the patient (Box 3.1). Harm associated with diagnosis is the commonest threat to patient safety in both primary and secondary care.

The extent of threats to patient safety associated with diagnosis

The exact frequency is unknown, because of different methods of identification, but the overall message remains. The level is unacceptably high.

Box 3.1 **Cascade of errors**

- A chain of errors (a cascade) occurred in 77% of patient safety incidents.
- Sixty-six percent of diagnostic errors were set in motion by errors in communication, either informational or personal communication.
- Examples of informational miscommunication included communication breakdowns among colleagues and with patients (44%), misinformation in the medical record (21%), mishandling of patients' requests and messages (18%) and inaccessible medical records (12%).

(After Woolf SH, Kuzel AJ, Dovey SM, Phillips RL. A string of mistakes: the importance of cascade analysis in describing, counting, and preventing medical errors. *Annals of Family Medicine* 2004;**2**:317–326.)

Box 3.2 **Analysis of 56 incidents relating to results**

- Arranging a test (e.g. labelling errors, sample lost in transit) 26.9%
- Testing process (e.g. wrong test performed, laboratory error) 19.2%
- Communication of test to GP (e.g. excessive delay or not sent) 17.3%
- Processing result (e.g. filed unseen, urgent test not shown to GP) 15.4%
- Communication to patient (e.g. GP forgot, patient given wrong result) 21.2%

(After Bhasale A, Norton K, Britt H. Tests and investigations. Indicators for better utilisation. *Australian Family Physician* 1996;**25**:680–694.)

Primary care

Fifty-four percent of all adverse events reported in medico-legal databases are the result of failure or delay in diagnosis, and 25% of all adverse events are due to a wrong diagnosis. The largest categories are malignant neoplasms and septicaemia, including meningococcal septicaemia. Other categories are diseases of the circulatory system, including chest pain and peripheral vascular occlusion, and injuries. There is often over-reliance on normal investigations and lack of appropriate examination.

Incident reporting of events that caused, or had the potential to cause, harm reveals that 53% are due to missed or delayed diagnosis. There is a range of causes (Box 3.2).

Secondary care

Twenty-one percent of all adverse events reported in medico-legal databases are the result of failure or delay in diagnosis.

Twenty percent of reviewed deaths are misdiagnosed, and 44% of these cases would have been treated differently if the correct diagnosis had been made.

Causes of threats to patient safety associated with diagnosis

Making a diagnosis in both primary and secondary care is not an easy task, especially when the presented problems are complex (Box 3.3).

Box 3.3 Common difficulties in making a diagnosis in both primary and secondary care

- Patients may present at an early stage of an illness when the symptoms and signs are ill-defined and vague.
- Patients (or their families) may present when they are at their limit of tolerance – due either to the level of symptoms or to their level of anxiety.
- Problems are often complex and a mixture of physical, psychological and social factors.

The diagnostic process

Taking a full history, examining the patient fully and performing a wide range of investigations are not only potentially wasteful of time and resources but do not guarantee that a correct diagnosis will be made; some investigations may actually harm the patient. Most of these aspects are dependent on effective communication between doctor and patient.

A diagnosis is made by generating and ranking appropriate diagnostic possibilities. The most important approach is to make an estimate of the likely cause, or causes, of the patient's symptoms. The potential seriousness of each of these possibilities is then considered, and also how amenable they are to treatment. For example, hypothyroidism is an uncommon cause of tiredness, is potentially serious but can be easily treated. Very rare and novel conditions are often considered, especially if there is previous personal experience of these conditions, but it is important that the applicability to the particular patient is considered (Box 3.4).

Problems in the diagnostic process

Making a diagnosis is complex, and there are many factors associated with problems in this process. Among the most common pitfalls are: maintaining a focus on a particular diagnosis, ignoring or not pursuing alternative hypotheses, and not ruling out competing hypotheses when they are very unlikely. This latter process often results in numerous investigations being performed. It is important to remember that a positive test when there is a low possibility of the disease is more likely to be a false-positive. This can lead to inappropriate, and possibly harmful, interventions (Boxes 3.5–3.7).

Doctor–patient communication difficulties in making a diagnosis

An essential aspect of making a diagnosis is effective communication so that a full history is obtained, the health beliefs of the patient

Box 3.4 Generation and ranking of diagnostic possibilities

- Probability
- Seriousness
- Treatability
- Rarity and novelty

(From Elstein AS, Shulman LS, Sprafka SI. *Medical Problem Solving – An Analysis of Clinical Reasoning*. Harvard University Press, Cambridge MA, 1978.)

Box 3.5 Common errors in making a diagnosis

- Unwarranted fixation on a hypothesis
- Premature closure of hypothesis generation
- Rule out syndrome

(From Joorabchi B. Medical information processing skills: guideposts to clinical assessment. *Medical Teacher* 1989;**11**:331.)

Box 3.6 Common factors other than disease that may influence diagnostic test results

- Age and sex
- Body position
- Chance phenomenon
- Laboratory error

Box 3.7 Common identified causes of errors in diagnosis

Human factors

Misdiagnosis can occur when the healthcare professional is tired or overworked. However, the reasons for this are related to underlying system factors.

System factors

- Assessment by insufficiently experienced staff
- Inadequate systems for recording findings
- Inadequate use of specialist opinion
- Inadequate reading of simple radiographs
- Poor management of routine situations, with lack of use of standard protocols and best practice guidelines
- Inadequate assessment before discharge

and carer are identified, and there is a shared understanding of the presented problem and the proposed management plan.

Cultural aspects in making a diagnosis

Individuals each have their own set of values and beliefs. Identification of these will help the healthcare provider to understand the individual and his or her unique perspective on the world. It will also reveal values and beliefs that are collectively held by a particular cultural group. It is important not to discount views that are different from those of the interviewer. The attribution of the symptoms by the patient may help in the diagnostic process, especially when the diagnosis is specific to a particular culture. It is always important to listen to what the patient, and carer, is telling the healthcare provider.

Difficulties associated with the use of telephone and e-mail consultations

The majority of consultations are still face-to-face but there are increasing numbers of consultations by telephone and e-mail. These consultations create difficulties with communication and can lead to major diagnostic errors. There is a lack of nonverbal cues, and the patient's condition and context cannot be easily determined. It is essential to be more vigilant when using these alternative methods of communication.

Causes of threats to patient safety associated with diagnostic results management

Over 70% of GP practices in risk reviews have identified results handling as a major risk area. Patients usually assume that their doctor will notify them of the result, but this is often not the case for a variety of reasons.

The process of performing even a simple diagnostic test is complex, and many people may be involved. The essential steps include taking the sample, processing the sample, processing the results and taking action. All of these steps are vulnerable and can result in a threat to patient safety. Particular care has to be taken for high-risk results, such as pregnancy tests and those used for monitoring treatment with drugs, such as lithium or anticoagulants.

It is good practice for all healthcare providers to establish effective systems for results handling. There is no foolproof system but important features include:

- Fully and legibly complete both the request form and the sample.
- Make a record of the result and set a review date.
- Reconcile each result received with the tests taken.
- Ensure that all abnormal results are seen by a doctor and that prompt actions are taken.
- Ensure clinical decisions or actions relating to the results are recorded in patients' notes.
- Inform patients of the results.
- Audit compliance with these actions regularly.

This advice is equally applicable to secondary care providers but the extent of these factors in secondary care is often unknown.

Causes of threats to patient safety associated with referrals

Referral from primary to secondary care is often an important part of the diagnostic process but it is a common cause of threat to patient safety, especially because there may be a lack of or delay in referral.

Referrals may be inadvertently lost, especially when there is a delay between the decision to refer and the actual referral letter being produced. The referral may be 'lost in the system'. In primary care, the 'referral system' can be complicated, with numerous steps between seeing the patient in primary care and the patient being seen in secondary care. It is hoped that the new national 'Choose and Book' programme in the UK will reduce these types of event.

An important cause of delay in referrals for serious illnesses, such as chest pain or suspected cancer, is lack of adherence to early referral guidelines – the urgent 'two-week referrals'. The early detection of many cancers can be difficult because the symptoms are often nonspecific, yet this is the most appropriate time for urgent referral. In the UK, the National Institute for Clinical Excellence (NICE) has recently published practical guidelines on the early detection and referral of several cancers, especially breast, lung and lower gastrointestinal tract.

Practical approaches to reducing adverse events associated with diagnosis

Several approaches can be taken that can reduce adverse events associated with diagnosis:

- Take a history that concentrates on the key elements.
- Assess the evidence and consider the possible range of differential diagnoses.
- Use diagnostic tests appropriately. It is important to be aware of the sensitivity and specificity of the screening test.
  - A test with a high sensitivity will have fewer missed diagnoses.
  - A test with a high specificity will have fewer false alarms.
  - A positive test when there is a low possibility of the disease is more likely to be a false-positive.
- Carefully consider whether discharge from care is appropriate.
- Obtain a second opinion if the problem remains unexplained.

Further reading

Black ER, Bordley DR, Tape TG, Panzer RJ. *Diagnostic Strategies for Common Medical Problems*, 2nd edn. American College of Physicians, Philadelphia, 1999.

Elstein AS, Schwarz A. Evidence base of clinical diagnosis: Clinical problem solving and diagnostic decision making: selective review of the cognitive literature. *Br Med J* 2002;**324**:729–732.

Heller R, Sandars J, Patterson L, McElduff P. GPs' and physicians' interpretation of risk, benefits and diagnostic test results. *Family Practice* 2004;**1**:155–159

Further resources

Massachusetts Coalition for the Prevention of Medical Errors has produced comprehensive guidance and a toolkit for communicating critical test results, which may be accessed at their website (www.macoalition.org/initiatives.shtml).

CHAPTER 4

Use of Medication

Darren M Ashcroft, Judith A Cantrill

OVERVIEW

- Medicines are the most commonly used clinical intervention
- Complications arising from the use of medicines are among the most common causes of adverse events in healthcare, both primary and secondary
- Threats to patient safety due to the use of medication can occur at all stages of the process, from the initial decision to prescribe to medication review
- Increased threats to patient safety due to the use of medication are found in the very young, the elderly, and patients on multiple medications

Medicines are the most commonly used clinical intervention. Every day, around 1.8 million prescriptions are written by general practitioners in England, with an additional 0.5 million prescriptions written in hospitals. Ensuring the safe and efficacious use of medicines is a challenging and complex process. It is an unavoidable fact that medicines that bring genuine benefit to patients will always carry some degree of risk. Even when used correctly, medicines can be associated with adverse outcomes.

Terminology

Adverse drug events, adverse drug reactions and medication errors have been defined in a variety of different ways. Some of the more commonly used definitions are shown in Box 4.1. An adverse drug event (ADE) refers to an injury caused by medication, such as gastrointestinal bleeding caused by nonsteroidal anti-inflammatory drugs (NSAIDs). Adverse drug reactions (ADRs) form a subset of ADEs that occur at recommended drug dosages. They are often categorized into two broad groups – those that can be predicted from knowledge of the drug's pharmacological effects on the body (Type A) and those that are unpredictable, idiosyncratic reactions that occur in particular individuals (Type B). Type A reactions are more common than Type B, accounting for over 80% of all reactions. Specific examples of ADRs include allergic reactions to aspirin when the allergy was unknown, or hair loss following a course of cancer chemotherapy. By contrast, medication errors may occur from the initial decision to prescribe to the final administration of the medi-

cine, and these include selection of the wrong medicine, dose, route and frequency or time of administration.

Figure 4.1 shows the relationship between ADEs, ADRs and medication errors. The relative sizes of each category will depend on the actual rate of ADEs and medication errors within any healthcare setting. ADEs may or may not result from medication errors – for example, an allergic reaction to flucloxacillin in a patient without a known history of penicillin allergy is not the result of a medication

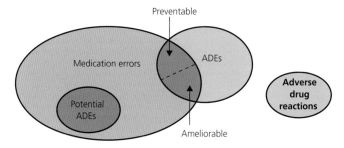

Figure 4.1 Relationship between adverse drug events (ADEs), adverse drug reactions and medication errors.

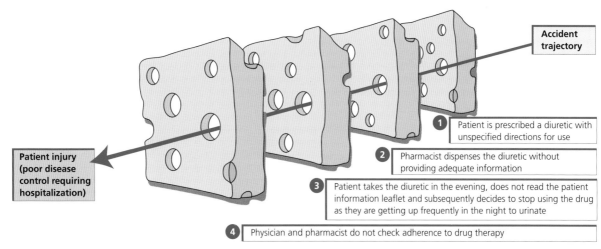

Figure 4.2 Reason's 'Swiss cheese' model applied to medication-related problems resulting in patient injury.

error, whereas a medication error has occurred if the patient had a prior history of penicillin allergy. By definition, medication errors are preventable. Where the error is recognized the situation can be retrieved (i.e. administration stopped) and no injury to the patient may occur; moreover, sometimes patients suffer no adverse consequences from receiving the wrong medication.

Nature and extent of threats to patient safety associated with medication in primary and secondary care

Complications arising from the use of medicines constitute one of the most common causes of adverse events in healthcare. Within four weeks of receiving a prescription in primary care, 25% of patients experience an ADE, 11% of which are judged preventable. Approximately 5% of all hospital admissions are associated with ADRs, with higher prevalence rates (11%) reported in studies of elderly patients. While in hospital, the oral drug administration error rate is approximately 5% of all doses due. The preparation and administration of intravenous drugs is also inherently risky; a UK study in two hospitals found errors in almost half of the drug doses observed, of which 1% of doses had potentially serious errors (Box 4.2).

Inadequate drug and patient knowledge and lack of timely access to information have been identified as important root causes of medication errors. Other risk factors include the work environment, workload, illegible prescriptions, poor communication and poor history taking. Organizational factors include inadequate training and low perceived importance of risks associated with medicines.

With long-term drug therapy, the most appropriate drug may be chosen and prescribed in the correct dose, frequency and duration. However, one of the commonest causes of adverse outcomes is failure to monitor. Repeat prescribing has been identified as an important source of error, especially in the absence of standard operating procedures. A study in UK general practice found that for 72% of repeat drugs prescribed, there was no evidence of a review by a doctor within the previous 15 months.

Reason proposed the 'Swiss cheese model' to illustrate how accidents can occur within systems. This analogy compares the defensive layers of the system to layers of Swiss cheese, each having holes that represent safety failures. The presence of holes in one slice may not result in an adverse event, because the other slices act as safeguards. However, the holes in the layers may temporarily line up, creating an opportunity for an accident. Figure 4.2 shows how multiple failures in the drug use process can result in patient harm (Figure 4.3).

Box 4.2 **The frequency and extent of errors associated with the use of medication in primary care**

- Potential adverse drug reactions identified in 0.13% of prescriptions.
- About 5% of admissions to hospital in UK due to an adverse drug reaction. The adverse reaction resulted in death in 2% of cases.
- Between 13% and 51% of all reported adverse incidents that occur in primary care are related to medication.
- About 20% of all claims identified on medico-legal databases are related to medication.

(After Sandars & Esmail, 2002.)

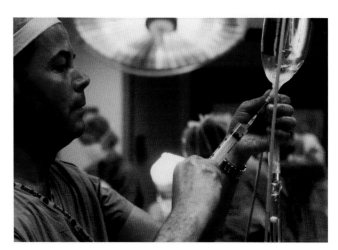

Figure 4.3 Intravenous drug infusion – a risky scenario! (Reproduced with permission of Michael Donne/Science Photo Library.)

Residential and nursing homes and transfer between settings

Medication errors may also arise when patients are transferred from primary care (own home, residential or nursing care) to secondary care. On average, two medication errors occur each time a patient is transferred from primary care, the most common error being inadvertent withdrawal of drugs. In contrast, when patients leave the hospital the most common problem is erroneous addition of drugs.

One of the most recent studies in long-term care facilities suggested that ADEs occur at the rate of approximately 9 per 100 resident months, half of which were judged to be preventable. More serious adverse events were also likely to be predictable. Drugs most commonly implicated include warfarin, antipsychotics, loop diuretics, opioids, antiplatelets and angiotensin-converting enzyme (ACE) inhibitors. The most frequent types of ADE were neuropsychiatric, haemorrhagic, renal/electrolyte and gastrointestinal problems.

How can threats to patient safety associated with the use of medication be reduced?

There are no easy solutions but there are some important approaches. The main areas to consider are:

- **The decision to prescribe.** A key issue in any prescribing decision is to balance possible risks and benefits. It may be that the safest option is not to prescribe or that further information is obtained about the drug or the patient. This includes considerations about the drug (such as cautions, contraindications, interactions and side effects) or about the patient (such as age, sex, presence of other diseases and allergies) (Box 4.3).
- **Medication reviews and monitoring.** Long-term medication should be reviewed because circumstances often change, such as the addition of further drugs or the development of new diseases. Repeat prescribing reviews are essential, especially in the elderly. The exact frequency of these reviews will depend on the drug being prescribed and the condition of the patient, both medical and social.
- **Patient education.** Discussion with patients will often identify their ideas about starting medication – they may not expect a drug. Patients should be encouraged to take an active part in reducing drug errors, such as reading patient information leaflets in the packaging.
- **Improvements to the design of medicine packaging could help improve medication errors.** It is estimated that a third of medication errors are caused by confusion over packaging and labelling instructions. The National Patient Safety Agency (NPSA) has

---

Box 4.3 Common reasons for errors occurring: the initial prescription

- Inadequate knowledge of the patient and their clinical condition
- Inadequate knowledge of the drug
- Calculation errors
- Drug name confusion
- Poor (clinical and medication) history taking

Box 4.4 Practical points to improve safety with long-term drug therapy

- Set therapeutic targets and time scales (e.g. by how much you want the blood pressure to fall and when do you expect this to happen).
- Warn the patient about the most predictable side effects. Explain whether these will: (i) decrease with time, (ii) persist, so that the patient needs to decide whether he or she can 'live' with them, or (iii) mean that the patient needs to inform the prescriber if they occur.
- Arrange appropriate follow-up (laboratory monitoring and/or consultation).
- At follow-up, assess both benefits (achievement of therapeutic targets) and risks (occurrence of unwanted effects).
- Set a new target and repeat the process.

---

published *Information Design for Patient Safety*, which shows how graphic design on medicine packaging can enhance patient safety. It is available from the NPSA website (www.npsa.nhs.uk).

Information gathered by the NPSA on medication errors has been used to help develop practical solutions and advice for the UK's National Health Service (NHS). These solutions are issued in the form of patient safety alerts, which require NHS organizations to address high-risk safety problems. Patient safety alerts relating specifically to medicines include advice on the safe use of morphine and diamorphine injections, methotrexate and childhood vaccines.

The simple advice is that before any drug is prescribed consider these questions: 'could this drug possibly harm this patient?'; and 'how can I minimize any possible harm?'. There are future considerations for long term drug therapy (Box 4.4).

Role of the pharmacist in reducing threats to patient safety associated with the use of medication

Pharmacists have traditionally played an important quality control role in checking patients' medication. In the UK, on average seven interventions are made by community pharmacists for every 1000 items dispensed. These result from a variety of reasons that reflect shortcomings in the basic rules of safe prescribing, such as selecting the wrong drug, dose, quantity or strength of medication, with higher error rates detected on handwritten prescriptions.

Likewise, hospital pharmacists detect errors in around 1.5% of prescription items. The majority of errors (54%) are associated with the drug dose, and most serious errors originate in the prescribing decision. Not surprisingly, both the experience of the pharmacist and the time that they spend on the hospital ward have been shown to be significant predictors of an increased error detection rate.

Role of information technology (IT)

Computing systems already exist that can link patient history, laboratory results and prescribing data and present a hierarchy of warnings to inform, advise and, in specific circumstances, prohibit the prescribing of medicines (Box 4.5). In the USA, research has shown

Box 4.5 **Ways that information technology can reduce errors**

- Improve communication
- Make knowledge more readily accessible
- Require key pieces of information (such as the dose of a drug)
- Assist with calculations
- Perform checks in real time
- Assist with monitoring
- Provide decision support

that the use of computerized physician order entry and decision support systems can substantially reduce the incidence of serious medication errors. Despite this, the adoption of IT initiatives to reduce risk associated with medicines has been limited. To date, studies have generally been conducted in specialized settings and rarely in primary care where the vast majority of prescribing takes place.

However, the safety of IT initiatives should not be taken for granted. Like other interventions designed to improve patient safety, there is a need to ensure that they are subject to rigorous evaluation before wholesale adoption into practice. Recent work has shown that the safety features of a large proportion of computing systems used in UK general practices have clinically important deficiencies, which may fail to warn prescribers in situations when warnings would be expected.

In addition, there are now a number of studies that have reported on prescribers switching off software-generated onscreen drug interaction alerts when writing prescriptions. In one UK study, a fifth of the general practitioners responding to a survey admitted to overriding drug interaction alerts without properly checking them. In the hospital setting, a UK study tracking elective surgical patients from preoperative assessment to discharge found that the majority of medication errors were detected at the stage of computerized prescribing of discharge medication.

Further reading

Audit Commission. *A Spoonful of Sugar: Medicines Management in NHS Hospitals*. Audit Commission, London, 2001.

Bates DW, Gawande AA. Improving safety with information technology. *N Engl J Med* 2003;**348**:2526–2534.

Berman A. Reducing medication errors through naming, labelling and packaging. *J Med Syst* 2004;**28**:9–29.

Cousins D. Safe medication initiatives – sustaining good practice. *Hospital Pharmacist* 2006;**13**:215–217.

Sandars J, Esmail A. *Threats to Patient Safety in Primary Care: A Review of the Research into the Frequency and Nature of Error in Primary Care*. Department of Health, London, 2002. (www.pcpoh.bham.ac.uk/publichealth/psrp/pdf/sanders_esmail_threats.pdf).

Smith J. *Building a Safer NHS for Patients: Improving Medication Safety*. Department of Health, London, 2004 (http://www.dh.gov.uk/PublicationsAndStatistics/Publications/PublicationsPolicyAndGuidance/PublicationsPolicyAndGuidanceArticle/fs/en?CONTENT_ID=4071443&chk=PH2sST).

Further resources

Institute for Safe Medication Practices (www.ismp.org).
National Patient Safety Agency (www.npsa.nhs.uk).
Saferhealthcare (www.saferhealthcare.org.uk).

Acknowledgement

We would like to thank Professor Carmel Hughes for providing data relating to residential and nursing homes.

CHAPTER 5

Communication and Patient Safety

Martin Beyer, Julia Rohe, Peter J Nicklin, Keith Haynes

OVERVIEW

- Communication problems with patients and within healthcare teams are a common cause of threats to patient safety
- Poor communication increases the potential risk of litigation
- Specific communication skills training can improve patient safety
- Adverse events are often due to communication difficulties across the interfaces of care

---

Communication is an essential part of the practice of medicine. It is also essential for patient safety. Communication is frequently a cause of, and a resource to prevent, threats to patient safety. The main areas for attention are communication with patients, within healthcare teams and across the various interfaces that occur within healthcare (Box 5.1).

Reports of adverse events, both actual and potential, from general practitioners in Germany identified that 15% of all events were related directly to problems of communication with carers and patients or within the team, and that in more than 50% communication was a contributing factor. Data from other studies are similar. In a study of Australian general practitioners, communication problems were one of the four main categories associated with adverse events, and this study also noted the importance of unclear medical records and problems associated with communication between various healthcare providers.

Analysis of available data, from both secondary and primary care, reveals that only one in eight patients claim against 'negligent'

Box 5.1 The scope of communication in patient safety

1 Communication is the basis to ensure the best process of care for the patient, to share aims and goals of care with the patient, and to share care with other professionals involved.
2 Communication in medicine often takes place under stress and time pressures.
3 Communication can help us to cope with situations of particular difficulty. Communication can improve collaboration in the team and with professional colleagues, to master uncertainty, and to avoid hazards to patient safety.

Box 5.2 Behaviours of doctors that increase the risk of a claim

- Desertion by the doctor. Something went wrong and the doctor was suddenly unavailable.
- Devaluing the views of patients and/or relatives.
- Delivering information poorly, or not at all.
- Failure to understand the perspective of the patient.

Table 5.1 Patient communication and the likelihood of malpractice claims

Doctors who had not been sued...[a]	Patients of doctors who were sued...[b]
- Asked patient questions - Explained the process of the consultation - Were perceived by patients to have spent sufficient time - Laughed	- Received no explanation - Felt ignored - Felt less time was spent - Felt rushed

[a]Source: Levinson W, Roter DL, Mullooly JP *et al.* Physician–patient communication: the relationship with malpractice claims among primary care physicians and surgeons. *JAMA* 1997;**277**:553–559.
[b]Source: Hickson GB, Clayton EW, Githens PB, Sloan FA. Factors that prompted families to file medical malpractice claims following perinatal injuries. *JAMA* 1992;**267**:1359–1363.

---

doctors, and it is not dependent on the level of technical expertise. The decision to make a claim appears to be related to how well the doctor had communicated with the patient and relatives, including explanation about the risks associated with investigation and treatment. If an adverse event does occur, effective communication can also reduce the likelihood of complaints and litigation (Box 5.2 and Table 5.1).

Communication problems and the patient

Research has highlighted the importance of communication, both verbal and nonverbal, to increase patient satisfaction with the consultation and compliance with the proposed management plan. This will also improve patient safety and reduce the likelihood of a complaint being made against the doctor. Longer consultations are associated with lower risk of malpractice claims, but it is important that the longer time is spent on effective communication. Communication problems are more likely when the doctor is in a hurry, angry or under stress. These are also the times when there is increased risk of adverse events.

It is essential to establish a relationship with the patient. Doctors should appear friendly, be polite and show that they are giving attention to their patient by allowing the patient to talk about their concerns. There is evidence that an unsatisfactory relationship can lead to the patient not giving sufficient information, and this can lead to problems with diagnosis and treatment.

The patient will often attend because of anxiety about their condition and with clear expectations about how it will be managed. The doctor should try to identify and understand the perspective of the patient. This can be difficult in patients with communication difficulties or where there are differences in social and cultural backgrounds.

Agreement about the presenting problem and its management plan has to be achieved. This requires sharing of information and negotiation. Common problems are the use of medical jargon and the lack of agreement by the patient about the management plan, especially if they do not understand what they have been told. It is essential to check patient understanding before the end of the consultation, including the arrangements for follow-up and when

---

Box 5.3 Examples of communication errors from the German Error Reporting and Learning System for General Practices (www.jeder-fehler-zaehlt.de)

Communication with the patient
The patient had a coronary artery stent and was discharged on several medications, including clopidogrel and aspirin. He was told to stop the clopidogrel after 4 weeks and to reduce the aspirin. He mistook the advice and stopped all medications, including an angiotensin-converting enzyme (ACE) inhibitor and beta-blocker.

Communication within teams
A patient in the surgery was supposed to receive 2 mg diazepam. The nurse misunderstood the verbal advice and gave 2 mL (10 mg). The patient became somnolent after he had received 5 mg i.v.

Communication across the interface of care
Due to an unclear hospital discharge prescription, the patient received only one-fifth of his usual dose of sodium valproate. He suffered a seizure as a result.

Box 5.4 Common problems in communicating with patients

- Lack of listening to or premature interruption of the patient's talk
- Use of medical terminology or jargon
- Lack of interest or compassion
- Lack of attention to the patient's views
- Disregard of communication handicaps of the patient (e.g. foreign language, hearing loss)
- Omission to verify that the patient understood the information presented
- Lack of time or availability to the patient

Box 5.5 Symptoms of disruptive communication behaviour

- Profane or disrespectful language
- Demeaning or offensive behaviour
- Sexual comments
- Lack of control of own emotions (e.g. anger)
- Criticizing staff in front of patients or co-workers
- Negative comments on care provided by others
- Inappropriate comments in case notes
- Dishonesty, lack of self-criticism, concealment of mistakes

(Adapted from Neff KE. Understanding and managing physicians with disruptive behavior. In: Ransom SB, Pinsky WW, Tropman JE (eds) *Enhancing Physician Performance: Advanced Principles of Medical Management*. American College of Physician Executives, Tampa FL, 2000, 45–72.)

Box 5.6 Identification of communication problems causing errors in systematic analysis of critical events: a checklist

- **Patient-related factors**
  Are there barriers to communication (language, understanding, attention)?
  Are there tensions in the doctor–patient relationship?
- **Task-related factors**
  Are laboratory results correctly communicated and understood?
  Are there protocols and procedures for handovers?
- **Individual factors of staff members**
  Are staff trained in communication skills?
- **Team factors**
  Do staff communicate effectively in the healthcare team?
  Are there problems with formal (written) communication, such as legibility of messages?
- **Workplace factors**
  Are there problems with workload, stress and frequent interruptions?
- **Organizational and management factors**
  Is there a culture of safety?
  Is there top-level commitment to adequate communication with the patients and within staff?

(Adapted from Taylor-Adams S, Vincent C. *Systems Analysis of Clinical Incidents. The London Protocol,* 2nd edn. Clinical Safety Research Unit, Imperial College London, 2004 (http://www.csru.org.uk/downloads/SACI.pdf).)

---

to seek help if the condition does not resolve or worsens (Boxes 5.3–5.6).

In the UK, the National Patient Safety Agency (NPSA) is encouraging patients and the public to become involved in patient safety issues through its 'Please Ask' campaign. At the heart of the campaign is making patients feel comfortable about asking questions about their National Health Service (NHS) healthcare and raising concerns with health professionals. This campaign includes a consumer magazine and Please Ask website (www.npsa.nhs.uk/pleaseask).

An NPSA guide to patient safety, *Seven Steps to Patient Safety*, offers detailed advice on developing ways to communicate openly with and listen to patients. It is available on the NPSA website (www. npsa.nhs.uk).

Communication about the risks of investigation and treatment

All healthcare interventions, whether for investigation or for treatment, carry a risk to the well-being of the patient. The assessment of risks by patients is primarily determined not by the facts but by the patients' emotions. Many complaints are made because the patient feels that the doctor was uncaring and that the risks were not explained so that the patient could understand them and make an informed decision.

There is now a substantial literature on how to communicate risk most effectively to give the patient greater satisfaction and certainty about making the best choice. Patients dislike descriptive terms, such as 'low risk', because it reflects the opinion of the doctor. The use of absolute numbers, combined with the presentation of both positive and negative outcomes, is preferred.

Throughout the process of communicating risk it is important to be honest about what is known, and not known, and to explore people's understanding, reactions and opinions about the information that they are given.

Communication after an adverse event

There is a tendency for doctors to reduce their communication with patients following an adverse event, especially because they often feel guilty and are anxious about the potential for a complaint or claim. Another barrier has been the widespread belief that saying sorry to patients and/or carers is an admission of legal liability; this is not true, but it has prevented clinicians from communicating effectively with patients and/or carers after an adverse event.

However, this is a crucial time when maintaining communication can help patients and carers to cope with the stress and trauma of being involved in an incident, and begin to rebuild trust between the patient and the healthcare team. There is tentative evidence from the USA that it may also reduce subsequent complaints and litigation claims.

It is important to be open after an adverse event. This can be shown by saying sorry for what has happened and by trying to help the patient understand what happened. The UK's National Patient Safety Agency (NPSA) has issued guidance on being open; this describes how to communicate effectively with patients and/or carers who have been involved in a patient safety incident. The NPSA has also developed training for clinicians and healthcare managers who have to hold *Being open* discussions with patients and/or carers. The *Being open* initiative has been widely supported by, amongst others, the Royal Colleges, the Medical Defence Union, the Medical Protection Society and the National Health Service (NHS) Litigation Authority. Further information is available from the NPSA website (www.npsa.nhs.uk).

Communication problems and teams

Communication within healthcare teams is mainly verbal but can also be written, such as the use of notes, message books and e-mail.

Box 5.7 The SBAR approach to communication in healthcare teams

First, the clinical staff need to state the **Situation**. Rather than 'Mr Jones is out of breath', the staff need to state 'The reason I am calling you is that Mr Jones in Room 301 is complaining of shortness of breath, which he states he has never had before.'

Second, is the **Background**: 'The background is, Mr Jones is a 57-year-old man who had abdominal surgery yesterday. He has no history of cardiac or lung disease.'

Third, is the **Assessment**: 'I've noticed that his breath sounds are decreased on the right side, he's having some pain, and I'm wondering if he has developed a pneumothorax.'

And fourth is the **Recommendation**: 'I think you need to come in and see him right now.'

There is further information about SBAR at the saferhealthcare website (www.saferhealthcare.org.uk).

Research in high-risk industries, such as aviation and petrochemicals, has highlighted the importance of communication to improve safety. Good communication in the team is essential, but the skills also include development of collective responsibility, resolution of differences between staff, and empowerment to speak out about observed problems in the safe operation of the various processes (Fig. 5.1). Airline staff are trained in techniques such as 'crew resource management', and similar approaches have started to be adopted for members of resuscitation and operating theatre teams.

A 'culture' of disruptive communication can develop, especially in hospitals, when the team is under stress and is constantly hurried. This culture of high emotional expression can lead to threats to patient safety. The importance of this aspect has been recognized in a proposed major patient safety goal of the Joint Commission on Accreditation of Health Care Organizations (US) for 2007.

A useful structure to employ when nurses, doctors or any member of the clinical team need to communicate about a patient's condition is SBAR –Situation, Background, Assessment and Recommendation Box 5.7).

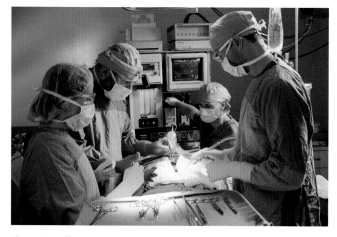

Figure 5.1 Effective communication is an essential part of teamwork. (Reproduced by courtesy of Getty Images.)

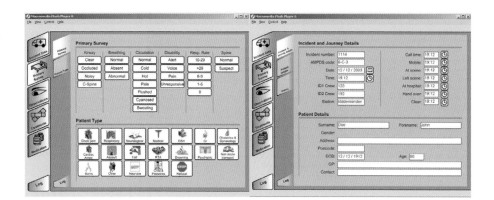

Figure 5.2 A clear interface improves communication. (Reproduced courtesy of Ortivus UK Ltd and Hereford and Worcester Ambulance Trust.)

Communication problems across the interfaces of care

All interfaces can lead to problems, whether they are between systems of healthcare, such as secondary and primary care, or between healthcare professionals, such as between doctors and nurses. Communication problems across interfaces are often identified as causes of, or contributing factors to, adverse events in systematic analyses of critical events.

Interfaces, of which there are large numbers in the typical healthcare context, are barriers that have to be crossed by effective communication. A variety of methods can be used, such as verbal messages, or documents, such as referral letters, discharge sheets or message books. In many countries, the procedures of referral, admittance or discharge from hospital have been improved by the use of electronic methods, and there is an expectation that 'electronic patient records' will be a solution (Fig. 5.2). However, there is still the need for personal communication with other healthcare providers, especially when the main barrier is often the different professional cultures.

Specific consultation skills training to reduce claims

Patients frequently judge the quality of medical care by the quality of communication they receive from their healthcare providers. In the USA and Australia medical insurers are sufficiently confident in the outcomes of communication skills training that they are a condition of a doctor's insurance or attract a substantial reduction in premium. An example of such a programme is that provided by the Medical Protection Society (MPS) in collaboration with the Cognitive Institute of Australia. The sessions concentrate on practising the ABCs of the clinical consultation – being Attentive, Benevolent and Compassionate. In particular, participants rehearse what is described as the 'golden minute', which includes greeting the patient, listening to the patient's story without interruption, and then summarizing the problem in an empathic manner. Critics of such training claim that it may merely protect the clinician against frivolous claims, but such interventions have a more serious intent: patients are reluctant to sue a doctor they like, and patients are less likely to comply with prescribed treatment if they do not feel their doctor has listened to them and understood their problem.

In conclusion, the challenge for the doctor is to be good not only at the clinical technical components of their work, but also at the interpersonal aspects. Communication is an essential skill that reduces both adverse events and also the likelihood of a complaint or a claim for negligence.

Further reading

Conradi M. *Oops ..., I'm so sorry! About Dealing with Mistakes and Complaints.* Nederlands Huisartsen Genootschap [Dutch College of General Practice], Utrecht, 2002 (http://nhg.artsennet.nl/upload/104/15524/c_a_7-e.pdf).

McTigue A. How to communicate with care. *UK Casebook* 2004;**12**:11–12 (http://www.medicalprotection.org/assets/pdf/casebook/casebook_2004_4_care.pdf).

Vincent C. Understanding and responding to adverse events. *N Engl J Med* 2003;**348**:1051–1056.

CHAPTER 6

Patient Safety Culture

Tanya Claridge, John Sandars

OVERVIEW

- The culture of an organization is increasingly being recognized as important for patient safety
- Each person in an organization has an individual, and a collective, responsibility for patient safety
- Development of a patient safety culture requires clear leadership of the organization
- Team-working approaches from aviation are useful methods to improve patient safety culture

All organizations have a culture – 'how things are done around here'. The organizational culture is often immediately apparent when an organization is encountered. For example, step inside any outpatient clinic and you will immediately receive an impression. Is it friendly? Are staff fraught? The culture comprises the shared attitudes, beliefs, values and assumptions that underlie how people within the organization go about their tasks. The same concept also applies to patient safety.

> The shared beliefs and values of the people who work within the organisation. This influences the way that people act in the organisation.

(From Kirk S, Marshall M, Claridge T *et al.* Evaluating safety culture. In: Walshe K, Boaden R (eds) *Patient Safety – Research into Practice.* Open University Press, Maidenhead, 2006, Chapter 13.)

Organizational safety culture

Research into high reliability organizations (HRO), which experience fewer accidents than expected, such as aircraft carriers and nuclear power plants (Fig. 6.1), has highlighted the importance of a culture of safety. Safety is the number one priority for the organization and for each of the workers that work within that organization. These organizations have several features:

- **High degree of autonomy but also interdependence.** Individuals are empowered to act as independent operators but rely on others to perform tasks.
- **Multiple cultures and teams that work interdependently.** Individuals work as part of cohesive teams, such as doctors or

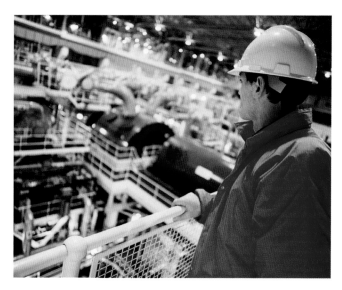

Figure 6.1 A nuclear powerplant as a HRO. (Reproduced courtesy of Getty Images.)

nurses, but also rely on other teams to achieve complex tasks effectively.
- **A prevailing attitude of chronic unease about potential safety threats.** There are formal rules and procedures but the purpose is to create 'heedful attention' to high-risk situations instead of routine compliance. There is usually one individual who takes an overall (executive) view of the situation and monitors the response to the situation.
- **Training is a high priority.** This includes clear required competencies that are regularly assessed, often by participating in simulations.
- **A collaborative structure takes over in situations of high risk.** In high-risk situations, the formal hierarchical relationships dissipate, all team members increase situational awareness, and each individual constantly monitors both the situation and the actions of other team members. Feedback on performance is freely given and received. The overall aim is to maintain safety.

Patient safety is as much about behaviour, values and attitudes as it is about physical action (Box 6.1).

The barriers to high reliability organizations in healthcare

A major barrier is blame apportioned to individuals for any adverse event. This is particularly common in healthcare, where there is a culture of high individual responsibility and where an error can lead to disciplinary or litigation proceedings. The response is that individuals tend to deny the possibility of error and are not willing to disclose adverse events because of the fear of possible recrimination.

The organization is often concerned with the wrong type of excellence. There may be management goals that are in pursuit of efficiency, cost savings or patient satisfaction, such as pleasant décor. The consequence is that patient safety is not expressed as a high priority.

Sociological studies of healthcare organizations have highlighted two further important issues that hinder the achievement of organizational goals and the maintenance of patient safety: division of labour and diffusion of responsibility.

Division of labour

Healthcare is complex and requires a differentiation of professional roles, such as doctors, nurses or social workers. The more complex the process, and the larger the organization, the greater the need for more healthcare workers of different types. This inevitably creates difficulties, with greater potential for errors to occur, because of the requirement to coordinate, collaborate and cooperate. Most healthcare workers have had different and separate training, and often hold a value system that is specific to their professional group.

Diffusion of responsibility

The problem of 'too many hands' involved in healthcare, especially when it is complex, results in a collective lack of responsibility for safety and little personal responsibility and feeling of accountability when adverse events occur.

Assessment of patient safety culture

An essential first step in the process of improving organizational culture is to assess its current state. There are only a few tools avail-able, and few have been developed specifically for healthcare, especially primary care. One such tool is the *Manchester Patient Safety Framework,* which has been adapted in collaboration with the National Patient Safety Agency (NPSA) for acute, mental health and ambulance settings. It is likely that further or refined tools will be developed in the future.

Most tools have two types of statement to represent the main safety culture dimensions – statements relating to values, beliefs and attitudes, and statements relating to behaviours that aim to improve safety, such as leadership, policies and procedures. These aspects are identified by the use of self-completed questionnaires (Box 6.2).

Developing a patient safety culture

The main challenge for improving safety is to achieve a cultural change. A recent survey of UK primary care managers noted that they regarded culture as an important concept but not one that they could predictably alter. However, patient safety can only be improved in partnership, and healthcare staff are key partners. The NPSA's Introduction to Patient Safety e-learning (IPSEL) is a programme that can help healthcare staff understand their role in improving patient safety. It is available at the NPSA website (www.npsa.nhs.uk/health/resources/ipsel).

An important first step is to ensure that patient safety is high on the list of priorities for the healthcare organization, and this needs to be coupled with a clear executive responsibility, not only at the top but also at each level of the organization, including each clinical team (Box 6.3).

Cultural change is concerned with how people feel and think about issues. Opportunities have to be created for people to freely state their opinions, and this openness then needs to be transferred to systems that allow all individuals to report and discuss adverse events. A 'no blame' culture gives individuals an opportunity to dis-

Box 6.3 **Developing a safety culture**

- Declare patient safety as a priority.
- Establish executive responsibility for patient safety.
- Import new knowledge and skills.
- Install a blameless reporting system.
- Develop accountability.
- Reform education and develop organizational learning.
- Accelerate change for improvement.

(After Morath JM, Turnbull JE. *To Do No Harm: Ensuring Patient Safety in Health Care Organizations*. John Wiley & Sons, San Francisco, 2005.)

close and discuss without fear of punishment, but it does not absolve individuals from being accountable for their actions. An important aspect of developing a safety culture is to ensure that each individual regards themself as being personally, and collectively, responsible for safety. Safety is everyone's concern.

Many incident reporting systems have faltered when it is apparent that the organization has not taken note of the comments and produced changes in the way that it performs. This requires the organization to have a willingness to learn from these incidents, no matter how trivial or at variance with its planned actions, and the changes have to be made demonstrable to the workers in the organization. It has to be seen that something has been done. The NPSA's *Seven Steps to Patient Safety* gives advice on how healthcare organizations can promote the reporting of patient safety incidents at a local and national level, and embed lessons through changes to practice, processes and systems. This guide is available from the NPSA website (www.npsa.nhs.uk).

Executive walk rounds (EWRs) are a widely used activity designed to improve safety culture in hospitals. A recent study concluded that EWRs have a positive effect on the safety climate attitudes of nurses

Box 6.4 **How will you know that culture has been changed in your organization or your team?**
- People will see that management/team leadership is committed to safety, by prevention not punishment.
- A healthy, happy staff is seen as an essential factor in safe care.
- Staff take their own health and well-being seriously as well as that of their colleagues, and can recognize when things are going wrong.
- Error and problems are anticipated by systems being proactive.
- Staff will consistently feel able to confront others about their unsafe acts; will report unsafe conditions; and will give priority to safety over efficiency.
- Staff and management will consistently implement remedial actions.
- Safety will be seen as essential and exciting.

(After Morath JM, Turnbull JE. *To Do No Harm: Ensuring Patient Safety in Health Care Organizations*. John Wiley & Sons, San Francisco, 2005.)

who participate in the sessions. EWRs are a promising tool to improve the safety climate and the broader construct of safety culture (Box 6.4).

> The biggest challenge to moving toward a safer health system is changing the culture from one of blaming individuals for errors to one in which errors are treated not as personal failures, but as opportunities to improve the system and prevent adverse events.

(Kohn LT, Corrigan JM, Donaldson MS (eds). *To Err is Human*. Institute of Medicine, Washington DC, 2001.)

Crew resource management approaches

The investigation of several major aviation accidents showed that cockpit errors occurred despite various procedures that were thought to increase safety, such as the use of checklists. The main factor associated with these accidents was inadequate communication between crew members, especially related to situational awareness, with the result that there was a breakdown in the possible organizational defences.

Crew resource management is not concerned with the technical skills but concentrates on the important cognitive and interpersonal skills required for safe operation. The main aspects are:

- **Situational awareness.** This requires constant awareness of the various factors – operational, technical and human – that affect safe operation. Individuals increase their awareness that under certain conditions error is more likely to occur, such as a delay in commencement of a procedure, working in a different environment, or when there is undue stress in any member of the team. The result is increased vigilance.
- **Planning and decision-making.** Roles are clearly defined and the respective areas of responsibility are identified. Potential high-risk situations are rehearsed.
- **Communication.** Effective communication between team members is essential. This not only includes making clear and unambiguous messages but also recognizes that making and receiving messages is dependent on a willingness to make the action.

Based loosely on simulator training in commercial aviation, there has been increasing use of surgical operating room training to increase patient safety. An example is Team Oriented Medical Simulation (TOMS), which allows an operating team, including all the healthcare workers involved in the surgical procedure, to explore new behaviours on the job, without risk to human life. These sessions consist of a preoperative training period, the simulation itself, and a debriefing of the simulation. Video recordings of the simulation are used to illustrate and reinforce training issues, especially those related to those aspects of crew resource management.

Overall, it is important to ask: 'How can I make this activity as safe as possible?' This is a responsibility for all members of the organization, from the healthcare workers to managers. Patient safety is a number one priority.

Further reading

Helmreich RL. On error management: Lessons from aviation. *Br Med J* 2000;**320**:781–785.

Morath JM, Turnbull JE. *To Do No Harm: Ensuring Patient Safety in Health Care Organizations.* John Wiley & Sons, San Francisco, 2005.

Musson DM, Helmreich RL. Team training and resource management in healthcare: Current issues and future directions. *Harvard Health Policy Review* 2004;**5**:25–35.

Thomas EJ, Sexton JB, Neilands TB *et al.* The effect of executive walk rounds on nurse safety climate attitudes: a randomized trial of clinical units. *BMC Health Serv Res* 2005;**5**:28.

Further resources

National Patient Safety Agency (NPSA). This has developed a wide range of guides, tools and training programmes. These are available on the NPSA website (http://www.npsa.nhs.uk).

Patient safety culture surveys

Hospital Survey on Patient Safety Culture (HSPC). Agency for Healthcare Research and Quality (http://www.ahrq.gov/qual/hospculture).

Manchester Patient Safety Assessment Framework (MaPSaF). National Primary Care Research and Development Centre, University of Manchester (http://www.npcrdc.man.ac.uk/ResearchDetail.cfm?ID=86).

Safety Climate Survey (SCS). University of Texas Centre of Excellence for Patient Safety Research and Practice (http://www.uth.tmc.edu/schools/med/imed/patient_safety/survey&tools.htm).

CHAPTER 7

Principles of Clinical Risk Management

Julie Price, Peter J Nicklin, Keith Haynes

OVERVIEW

- Risk is an inevitable part of life and cannot be absolutely removed, but it can be minimized
- All aspects of the healthcare process are associated with clinical risks
- Management of clinical risks should be proactive and use planned systems to prevent or reduce potential risks
- Clinical risk management can be reactive and respond to identified risks or potential risks

Risk, 'the possibility of incurring a misfortune or loss', is a normal part of daily life. We are constantly exposed to a wide variety of hazards, whether crossing the road or working in the kitchen, and we spend a large proportion of each day in attempts to avoid the possibility of an accident, injury or other misfortune. Anticipating hazards and reducing the likelihood of a problem is risk management.

Principles of clinical risk management

It is often considered that all risks can be avoided, but this is an unrealistic and negative view. A more positive and alternative view is that risk has a constant presence but it can be managed by appropriate risk management processes. In the past, clinical risk management tended to be reactive, responding to adverse incidents, but there is now increasing emphasis for it to be proactive, in which risk is anticipated and accepted but appropriately managed (Box 7.1).

Box 7.1 Main steps in the clinical risk management process

- *Identify the risk* – what could possibly go wrong?
- *Analyse the risk* – what are the chances of it going wrong, its impact, and does it matter?
- *Control the risk* – is there anything you can do about it?
- *Cost the risk* – and if so, what is the cost of getting it right versus the cost of getting it wrong?
- *Record your findings and actions to be taken*
- *Monitor and review your risk assessment* – ongoing review is essential to ensure that your risk assessment stays up to date.

There are a number of key principles that underpin good clinical risk management, and these are related to the approaches taken by the healthcare organization to improve patient safety.

- There is a culture that values clinical risk management activities. Safety becomes a major priority for the organization.
- Systems for clinical risk management and quality assurance are interlinked. Despite a tendency to develop separate systems, high-quality care that is effective and efficient is also safe care. Separation can result in different priorities for resource allocation and attention by healthcare workers.
- The organization recognizes both collective and individual responsibility for managing clinical risk. Many healthcare organizations blame individual healthcare workers for adverse events, but the majority of adverse events are due to failures in the systems of care and are largely preventable. Blaming the individual avoids recognizing much wider problems in the organization and the subsequent taking of responsibility by the organization.
- There is a culture of accountability, but not blame, with support for those involved in patient safety incidents. Blaming individuals further demoralizes healthcare workers who are already blaming themselves for the adverse event. This can lead to reluctance to report adverse events. The alternative approach is to ensure that everyone reports all adverse events and learns from the event without the fear of reprisal.

Resources are made available to respond to identified clinical risks. It is important that once risks are identified they can be appropriately treated. A common reason for reduced motivation to report adverse events is the lack of any resultant action (Fig. 7.1 and Boxes 7.2–7.8).

The clinical risk management process

The clinical risk management process is about the planning, organization and direction of a programme that will identify, assess and ultimately control risk. The process can be represented by a sequence of steps but there is much overlap and often there is integration between all of the steps (Box 7.9).

Step 1: Establishing the context

The underlying reasons for managing clinical risk will determine how these risks will be managed. This context will include financial, political or legal aspects. There is usually a wide variety stakehold-

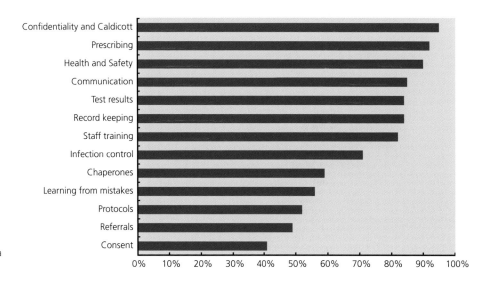

Figure 7.1 Risks in UK general practice. (Data supplied by MPS Risk Consulting, 2006.)

Box 7.2 **Confidentiality**

Ninety-five percent of UK general practices had risks associated with maintaining confidentiality:
- breaches of confidentiality in waiting rooms and reception areas;
- issues relating to Caldicott Guardians and Caldicott principles;
- staff contracts did not include a clause covering confidentiality post-employment;
- not all patient identifiable information was shredded;
- shredders were not always available;
- patient medical records were not securely stored;
- computers could be left on and unattended.

(Data supplied by MPS Risk Consulting, 2006; see Fig. 7.1.)

Box 7.3 **Health and safety**

Ninety percent of practices did not fully comply with all Health and Safety legislation (Health and Safety at Work Act 1974).

Areas of concern
- No health and safety assessment undertaken
- No Control of Substances Hazardous to Health (COSHH) assessment
- No personal protective clothing available
- Specimen handling
- Storage of clinical waste
- Storage of hazardous waste
- Storage of medication
- Issues related to sharps containers (Fig. 7.2)
- Issues related to spillage of bodily fluids
- Unlocked doors
- No panic alarms/protocols
- Security of prescription pads
- No VDU work station assessments
- Safety checks for small electrical items
- Unsafe furniture/fittings
- Cramped premises

---

ers, each with a different requirement. It is essential to identify these requirements and respond appropriately, since most will be required for accreditation or to satisfy a risk insurer. An example is the response required to the NHS Litigation Authority's General Clinical Risk Management Standards.

Step 2: Identification of risk

There are several methods that can be used to identify clinical risks, and these methods are usually performed in combination. The logic is that once adverse events have been identified they can be appropriately managed (Box 7.10).

One such method is the patient safety risk assessment process developed by the National Patient Safety Agency (NPSA) to support general practices, clinicians and local (integrated) commissioning groups when undertaking practice-based commissioning.

The usual approach is to consider adverse events after they have occurred. For example, a risk associated with the use of a particular medication could be identified by adverse events reported by healthcare workers, from complaints by patients or from compensation payments.

Each method will identify a different aspect of the frequency and nature of the risk. It can be expected that adverse events that result in compensation will be more severe and less frequent than those

associated with incident reports or complaints. Reliance on only one method will lead to errors in understanding the adverse event, either underestimating or overestimating its importance.

Risks can also be anticipated by creating a worst case scenario. In this approach it is often useful to construct a map that marks the main points on the pathways of the process of care. For example, it is possible to consider the main risks associated with a new surgical procedure by identifying the main steps in the pathway of care and then envisage the possible adverse events at each step, however rare they may be. This may identify critical points on the care pathway, such as the transfer from the operating theatre to the postoperative recovery area

The range of possible risks is usually very large, and it is not possible to identify all risks, especially since many are not obvious until

Box 7.4 **Prescribing**

Ninety-two percent of practices had risks associated with prescribing:
- no repeat prescribing protocol;
- no designated receptionist to record or generate repeat prescriptions – these are generated in the reception on an ad hoc basis, i.e. when time permits throughout the day;
- reception staff are allowed to add medication to the computer – acute and repeat medications;
- medication reviews are undertaken on an ad hoc basis. No review dates are set on the computer;
- there is no system for recalling patients on long-term medication, e.g. lithium, thyroxine or anticonvulsants;
- uncollected prescriptions are destroyed. It is not known what happens to prescriptions not collected from the pharmacy.

(Data provided by MPS Risk Consulting 2006; see Fig. 7.1)

Box 7.5 **Communication**

Eighty-five percent of practices had risks associated with communication issues within their practices:
- no regular practice meetings;
- no primary care meetings;
- some practices use 'Post-it' notes to pass messages within the practice, which are easily lost.

(Data supplied by MPS Risk Consulting, 2006; see Fig. 7.1)

Box 7.6 **Staff training**

Eighty-three percent of practices identified staff training needs:
- health and safety including fire;
- infection control and decontamination of instruments;
- Caldicott and confidentiality;
- learning from events;
- equipment use;
- repeat prescribing;
- management of violent/aggressive patients;
- communication skills;
- dispensing;
- emergencies;
- handling test results;
- annual resuscitation and anaphylaxis for all staff.

(Data supplied by MPS Risk Consulting, 2006; see Fig. 7.1)

Box 7.7 **Record keeping**

Eighty-four percent of practices had risks associated with record keeping within their practices:
- home visit consultations not always recorded on the computer;
- illegible writing in the records;
- letters scanned onto computer occasionally saved into the wrong record;
- telephone advice not always recorded;
- medical records go missing.

(Data supplied by MPS Risk Consulting, 2006; see Fig. 7.1)

Box 7.8 **Test results**

Eighty-four percent of practices had risks associated with test results within their practices:
- no tracker system to ensure that patients are followed up;
- no system of knowing when all a patient's test results have been returned;
- test results not recorded onto the computer;
- nonclinical staff allowed to inform patients of their result and the treatment required.

(Data supplied by MPS Risk Consulting, 2006; see Fig 7.1)

a new approach to diagnosis or treatment has been used for a period of time. This emphasizes the importance of adverse event incident reporting. However, it is usually possible to identify the most common or serious risks by worst case scenarios, with the result that appropriate risk reduction strategies can be implanted.

Step 3: Analysis of risk

Once a clinical risk has been identified, it should be analysed to determine what action needs to be taken. Ideally the risk should be eliminated, but usually this is not feasible and efforts are made to try to reduce it.

The potential probability and the potential impact (seriousness) of harm have to be considered. Decisions have to be made about a risk that is rare, but potentially very serious, compared with a risk that is very common but has a low probability to cause harm (Box 7.11).

A clinical risk that is rare but serious, such as a blood dyscrasia associated with a particular medication, has to be considered against a risk that is very common but less serious, such as a mild allergic skin rash with a different medication. It may not be possible to

Box 7.9 **Benefits of conducting a risk assessment**

- Improves the practice systems and quality of care provided
- Supports the practice development plan
- Useful evidence for appraisal and revalidation
- Reduces the likelihood of complaints and claims
- Improves communication within the team
- Assists in meeting the quality indicators of the new GMS contract and other regulatory requirements

Box 7.10 **Main approaches to the identification of a clinical risk**

- Incident reports of adverse events or near misses
- Review of clinical care records
- Direct observations of clinical care
- Complaints from patients
- Litigation and compensation claims and payments
- Interviews and questionnaires from patients and healthcare workers
- Routine data on clinical performance to identify unusual patterns, such as case mortality

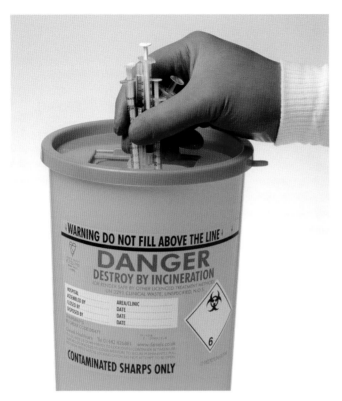

Figure 7.2 Safe disposal of sharps reduces the risk of needle-stick injury. (Reproduced by permission of Paul Rapson/Science Photo Library.)

predict who will experience the dyscrasia or to eliminate it, and so it has to be accepted. However, high numbers of mild adverse events may be regarded as a major risk and unacceptable, with the result that this medication is avoided unless its use is absolutely necessary.

Step 4: Treatment of risk

A range of choices are available to handle any identified clinical risk. The decision is mainly determined by the financial cost of implementation of treatment of the risk and the potential cost of compensation in the event of an adverse event. The cost of preventing one major, but very rare, adverse event may be very great when compared with preventing thousands of more minor adverse events.

- **Risk control.** It is not possible to eliminate all risks entirely but preventative steps can be introduced that minimise the likelihood

---

Box 7.11 **Factors to be considered in the analysis of a clinical risk**

- Probability of an adverse event happening
- Costs of an adverse event if it occurred (financial and other)
- Availability of methods to reduce the possibility of an adverse event happening
- Costs of possible solutions to minimize the adverse event (financial and other)

---

of an adverse event ocurring through the use of and adherence to guidelines, protocols and care pathways. For example, the use of guidelines for thromboprophylaxis in the perioperative period to reduce the risk of deep vein thrombosis and pulmonary embolus.

- **Risk acceptance.** This involves the recognition that the risk cannot be entirely removed but at least it can be known and anticipated. An example is the inevitable risk of failure for any equipment device, such as an infusion pump, and the provision of a back-up device in the event of a breakdown.
- **Risk avoidance.** It may be possible to avoid the risk by understanding the causes of the risk and taking appropriate actions. An example is the recognition that different medications may be packaged in identical ways, such as potassium chloride and sodium chloride ampoules (Fig. 7.3). This risk can be reduced by using packaging that clearly distinguishes the different medications.
- **Risk reduction or minimization.** Various strategies to reduce the risk are developed to limit the potential consequences of a given risk, with the acknowledgement that the risk cannot be avoided. This is the main approach to clinical risk management and includes training (both healthcare workers and patients) and policies and procedures. An example is the reduction in prescribing of inappropriate medication by the use of clinical guidelines and training.
- **Risk transfer.** This involves moving the risk of loss to another entity. This might be by transferring high risk and complex cases to a specialist centre. Or in situations where risk where risk cannot be easily mananged the risk of loss is covered by insurance.

Step 5: Evaluation of risk management process

In this step the effectiveness of the approaches used to identify, analyse and treat risks is reviewed. The role of audit is essential, in which risk management standards are set and monitored to see if these standards have been met. When problems are identified it is important to have a 'low-blame' culture so that people can honestly give their opinion of the cause and offer suggestions on how it can be reduced in the future. It is useful to have a multiprofessional approach, including patient representatives, since most adverse events have multiple causal factors, and a wide perspective is required for adequate identification and rectification (Boxes 7.12 and 7.13).

The complexity of clinical risk management

There is sometimes no simple or single method to reduce clinical risks. It is important to have increased vigilance and awareness of the increased likelihood of the possible occurrence of an adverse event. This is an essential feature of high reliability organizations in which adverse events rarely occur despite the background high risk of an adverse event. Clinical risk management should be both reactive, responding to adverse events, but also proactive to anticipate and prevent adverse events.

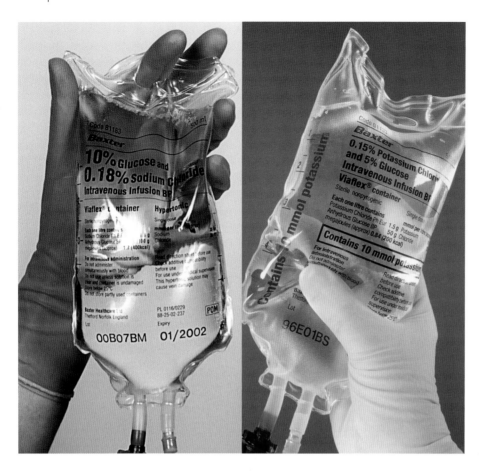

Figure 7.3 Clearly marked packaging can reduce risk. (Potassium chloride image reproduced by permission of Claire Paxton and Jacqui Farrow/Science Photo Library. Sodium chloride image reproduced by permission of Josh Sher/Science Photo Library.)

Box 7.12 Key requirements for a successful clinical risk management process

- Leadership with a commitment to improving patient safety
- Clear policy and strategy
- Organizational culture that regards patient safety as an important issue and that is accountable but blame free
- Incident reporting system that is accepted and regularly used
- Adequate resources to support the process and to respond to identified concerns
- Evaluation to ensure that the clinical risk management process is working

---

Box 7.13 Example of a clinical risk management strategy to reduce the risk of wrong site surgery

- Clinical risk standard introduced that provides context and increased awareness
- Training of all staff involved to develop increased awareness of the nature and frequency of wrong site surgery
- Development and use of a preoperative protocol
- Adverse event incident reporting analysed to identify frequency of wrong site surgery
- Regular review to evaluate the effectiveness of strategy

Further reading and resources

British Medical Association. Patient Safety and Clinical Risk – BMA Discussion Paper, December 2002 (http://www.bma.org.uk/ap.nsf/Content/patient-safetyclinicalrisk).

Haynes K, Thomas M. *Clinical Risk Management in Primary Care.* Radcliffe Medical Publishing, Oxford, 2005.

Kuyn AM, Younbberg BJ. The need for risk management to evolve to assure a culture of safety. *Quality and Safety in Health Care* 2002;**11**:158–162.

Medical Protection Society. MPS Risk Consulting website (clinical risk management resources) (http://www.mps-riskconsulting.com/content/).

National Patient Safety Agency website (http://www.npsa.nhs.uk/).

CHAPTER 8

Learning from Threats to Patient Safety

Maureen Baker, Richard Thomson, John Sandars

OVERVIEW

- Learning from threats to patient safety requires the collection and analysis of incidents
- Threats to patient safety are under-reported
- Root cause analysis and significant event audit provide structured approaches to understanding why threats to patient safety occur
- Local and national incident reporting systems provide widespread organizational learning from threats to patient safety

A necessary contribution to improving safety is the reporting of incidents; this usually involves healthcare staff recording information on events that have led to unintended harm or potential harm to patients. Incident reporting by itself cannot improve the safety of patient care; it is the learning from reporting that is critical. Such learning should be disseminated and implemented to help prevent the same problems occurring in future, ideally throughout a healthcare system.

Approaches to the collection and analysis of incidents

In the UK there are a number of hospital- and trust-wide (including primary care trusts, mental health and ambulance trusts) local risk management systems (LRMS) that support the collection and analysis of data on incidents. In addition, it is not uncommon for there to be more localized reporting systems in specific clinical settings, for example in pathology or intensive care.

There has been the development of national systems to capture incidents and promote wider learning. In the UK, the National Reporting and Learning System (NRLS) of the National Patient Safety Agency (NPSA) collects reports from across England and Wales, largely from LRMS (Fig. 8.1). The NRLS data set covers: free text description of what happened; when and where it happened; characteristics of the patient(s) involved; the outcome for the patient; and the staff involved in the incident and/or making the report. The data set also includes contributory factors and factors that might

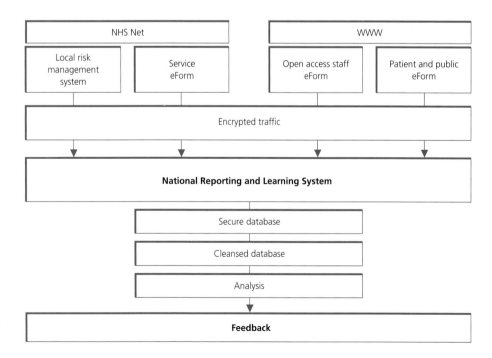

Figure 8.1 The National Reporting and Learning System. (Reproduced by permission of the National Patient Safety Agency.)

have prevented harm, but does not collect detailed information obtained from incident investigation. The NRLS approach contrasts with reporting systems that collect data following investigation, rather than at notification (such as the Joint Commission on Accreditation of Health Care Organizations (JCAHO) sentinel event system in the USA). A strength of the NRLS model is that reporters do not need to report twice, and that data on incidents from all settings are collected, but detail on individual incidents is more limited than in systems that collect extensive data from investigations (Box 8.1).

Improving incident reporting

Incident reporting systems are as good as the data collected and the use made of them. There are known limitations. Incident reporting systems are not comprehensive, because of under-reporting, biases in what types of incident are reported, and the existence of several reporting systems. Certain staff groups may report less than others (e.g. doctors less than nurses); certain incidents are more likely to be reported (e.g. falls rather than diagnostic errors); people are more likely to report if they can see action arising and if feedback occurs; and people are less likely to report if they perceive that they may be blamed.

The main approaches to improving incident reporting are prompted by being part of a supportive peer group that has raised awareness of patient safety, and by computers that have reminders, especially at crucial times for patient safety, such as on transfer or discharge from hospital.

Understanding why threats to patient safety happen

When things go wrong in healthcare, it is important to understand **why** and **how** things went wrong, and far less important (save in rare cases such as criminal activity or wilful negligence) to allocate blame. If there are underlying problems with the systems of care then similar events may happen again, only with different healthcare staff at the end of the sequence of events each time. There are a number of techniques that facilitate an understanding of why and how an incident happened, such as the NPSA's *Incident Decision Tree* framework. The framework can help staff be reassured that they will be treated fairly because it helps managers to take fair and consistent action when things go wrong.

Root cause analysis (RCA)

RCA describes a variety of methods that support more detailed retrospective investigation of selected incidents in order to understand better the factors that influenced the incident (not only contributing factors, but also protective factors that may have prevented harm occurring) (Box 8.2).

RCA is a suitable technique to be applied by healthcare organizations when a serious patient safety incident has occurred resulting in significant harm or death to a patient or number of patients. It might also be applied when an incident has affected a large number of patients, such as a large group of schoolchildren being administered an incorrect immunization. RCA is not feasible, nor appropriate, for all incidents; those leading to death or severe harm should justify an RCA, but it is also worth reviewing potentially severe incidents that were prevented (so-called near misses), since learning from these may be critically important in developing solutions. It is normally organized at management level by staff with the training and experience to conduct the analysis, and can involve many staff from within an organization, or sometimes from across organizations. RCA is usually an intense process that may take many hours, or even days, to complete. It potentially gives unparalleled depth of understanding of an incident. However, RCA needs to be undertaken in a skilled and structured way using a range of techniques. It needs to be ap-

Root Cause Analysis

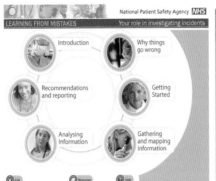
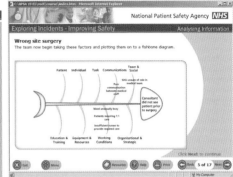

Figure 8.2 NPSA training on RCA. (Reproduced by permission of the National Patient Safety Agency.)

plied with sensitivity and care, and those using the technique need to be cognizant of its limitations. For example, retrospective methods are prone to recall bias; the first step in minimizing this is to be aware of it. Furthermore, as with incident reporting, RCA will only be effective if the findings are acted upon.

Training in how to carry out a root cause analysis is available from the National Patient Safety Agency's website (www.npsa.nhs.uk) (Fig. 8.2).

Significant event audit (SEA)

This technique is commonly used in the primary care sector, especially in general practice. It is normally conducted at practice, unit or team level, and a significant event can be either an adverse event or something that went really well – it should be possible to learn from excellence as well as from error. Like RCA this is a multidisciplinary activity, but SEA does not cover an event in the same detail as RCA (Box 8.3).

The role of SEA in patient safety is to view the process as a 'mini'-incident-reporting system in which adverse incidents are identified, made sense of and then actions taken to prevent similar occurrences in the future.

SEA and RCA are not mutually exclusive techniques. In fact one possible outcome from an SEA meeting may be to refer an incident to organizational level for consideration on whether an RCA should be conducted. Both these techniques should also be integrated with reporting mechanisms within healthcare organizations. All incidents should be reported, either locally or nationally, and one consequence of reporting might be to consider whether incidents should be further explored using SEA or RCA.

It is essential to consider certain logistic factors before introducing a significant event programme, especially leadership of the process. The ideal leader should be a person whom everyone respects and trusts. They should be enthusiastic for the process but be careful not to dominate the process. It is important to ensure that the meeting is at a time and place that is convenient for all team members. Many

> **Box 8.3 A structured process for significant event audit (SEA)**
>
> 1 Consider significant events for audit
> 2 Collect data on these events
>   • Identification of events for analysis
>   • Recording details of cases
> 3 Hold a meeting to discuss the events
>   • Implications of events
>   • Discussion of cases
>   • Decisions about cases
>   – immediate action
>   – no change in practice
>   – congratulations
>   – perform conventional audit
>   • Follow-up of cases
> 4 Documentation
> (From Sandars, 2005)

practice staff are part-time, including general practitioners. Some practices arrange meetings as part of the regular practice meeting, others hold separate meetings. A strength of significant event audit is the multidisciplinary aspect with all of the team present. However, it is important to remember that many practices have a large extended primary health care team that includes practice employed and attached staff (Boxes 8.4 and 8.5).

Maximizing patient safety information

Incident investigation techniques, together with incident reporting systems, provide the foundation for learning when things go wrong, but other sources of data may be required if the healthcare system as a whole is to learn from all types of incidents. Each healthcare organization should have a surveillance and monitoring approach that integrates data from a range of sources. The NPSA has set up a Patient Safety Observatory (PSO) in collaboration with a number of key national organizations, such as the Healthcare Commission, which is the independent regulator of health services in England; the Office for National Statistics; the Medicines and Healthcare Products Regulatory Agency, which regulates medicines and medical devices in the UK; patient organizations such as Action Against Medical Accidents; and the NHS Litigation Authority and other medical defence organizations. The primary function of the PSO is to quantify, characterize and prioritize patient safety issues

in order to support the NHS in making healthcare safer (Fig. 8.3 and Box 8.6).

   The PSO enables the NPSA to draw upon a wide range of data and intelligence, as a basis for identifying and monitoring patient

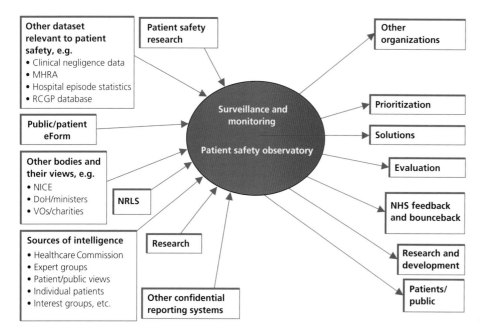

Figure 8.3 Root cause analysis. (Reproduced by permission of the National Patient Safety Agency.)

Box 8.7 **Analysis of critical incidents**

This is often called root cause analysis (RCA). It is essential that this has a multiprofessional approach since different people will usually offer a range of opinions.

The 'root cause' is the underlying cause in the system that produces the problem. If the root cause is identified and managed it should not recur.

Step 1: What happened?
It is important to list the various activities that occurred in the process of providing care. Often putting these details into a time sequence is helpful. For example, a near miss associated with drawing up a syringe of medication may be attributed to an unexpected admission on the ward, an inexperienced member of staff and a badly labelled drug ampoule.

There is usually a combination of factors that led to the event. Individuals should not be blamed for any actions.

Step 2: Why did it happen?
Consider all of these contributory factors:
- Organization and management
  Financial constraints
  Organization structure
  Safety culture
- Work environment
  Staffing levels and skills mix
  Workload and shift patterns
  Design, availability and maintenance of equipment
  Administrative and managerial support
- Team factors
  Communication
  Leadership
- Individual (staff) factors
  Knowledge and skills
  Physical and mental health
- Task factors
  Task design
  Use of protocols
  Availability of test results
- Patient factors
  Level of complexity and seriousness
  Communication
  Personality and social factors

Step 3: What are the specific and general contributory factors?
This step is concerned with identifying the specific factors directly associated with the event and more general factors that need to be considered.

It is important to identify any positive actions that were taken to prevent, or limit, harm.

Step 4: Feedback of the findings
A report that highlights several main recommendations for changes in the process of providing care is essential. All individuals, and the healthcare organization, can learn from the experience and begin to make changes to prevent further events in the future.

safety incident trends, highlighting areas for action and setting priorities. Incident reporting is considered alongside, for example, the published literature, clinical experts, medical record reviews, hospital episode statistics, death certification data, complaints, prospective risk assessments, patient safety indicator studies, observational research, confidential enquiries, and audits and reviews of healthcare organizations. Triangulating information from different data sources enables a fuller picture of the nature and severity of patient safety incidents to be obtained. The same approach is required within a local healthcare organization. Thus, as well as an LRMS, a hospital is also likely to: have data collected in local audits and morbidity/mortality meetings; provide reports to national confidential enquiries; collect data on complaints and litigation claims, and on patient diagnoses and adverse events within its patient administration system. Bringing these together under the wing of clinical governance is likely to be more powerful than relying on incident reports alone (Box 8.7).

Further reading

Barach P, Small SD. Reporting and preventing medical mishaps: lessons from non-medical near miss reporting systems. *Br Med J* 2000;**320**:759–763.

Department of Health. *An Organisation with a Memory: Report of an Expert Group on Learning from Adverse Events in the NHS.* Stationery Office, London, 2000.

Giles S, Fletcher M, Baker M, Thomson R. Incident reporting and analysis. In: Walshe K, Boaden R (eds) *Patient Safety – Research into Practice.* Oxford University Press, Oxford, 2006.

National Patient Safety Agency. *Seven Steps to Patient Safety.* NPSA, London, 2004.

National Patient Safety Agency. Building a Memory: Preventing Harm, Reducing Risks and Improving Patient Safety. The first report of the National Reporting and Learning System and the Patient Safety Observatory, NPSA, July 2005 (www.npsa.nhs.uk).

Sandars J. Significant event audit. In: Haynes K, Thomas M (eds) *Clinical Risk Management in Primary Care.* Radcliffe Medical Press, Oxford, 2005, 363–372.

Sandars J, Esmail A. *Threats to Patient Safety in Primary Care: A Review of the Research into the Frequency and Nature of Error in Primary Care.* Department of Health, London, 2002 (www.pcpoh.bham.ac.uk/publichealth/psrp/pdf/sanders_esmail_threats.pdf).

Vincent C, Taylor-Adams S, Stanhope N. Framework for analysing risk and safety in clinical medicine. *Br Med J* 1998;**316**:1154–1157.

World Health Alliance for Patient Safety. WHO *Draft Guidelines for Adverse Event Reporting and Learning Systems: from Information to Action.* WHO, Geneva, 2005 (http://www.who.int/patientsafety/events/05/Reporting_Guidelines.pdf).

Further resources

National Patient Safety Agency. Root cause analysis e-learning programme (www.saferhealthcare.org.uk/IHI/Products/E-learning/rcatoolkit.htm).

CHAPTER 9

Patient Safety and the Law

Michael Jones, Gary Cook

OVERVIEW

- It is estimated that more than 85 000 negligent adverse events occur each year in English hospitals; however, only around 6000 new medical negligence claims are dealt with each year
- In 2005–2006 clinical negligence claims cost the NHS £560 million pounds
- Medical or clinical negligence claims often originate from a failure to provide an adequate explanation or apology
- The Bolam test for negligence sets an objective standard of reasonable care, which is normally measured by reference to the relevant professional standards
- Inexperienced professionals should seek to have their work checked by a more senior colleague to avoid liability

The practice of medicine is covered by many legal sources. Both British and European conventions, statutes and statutory regulations comprise legal rules governing the practice and safe conduct of medicine. However, as Margaret Brazier points out in her book *Medicine, Patients and the Law*, much English law is made by judges, (common law), and is based on decisions and judgments handed down by the courts. The precedents set by this process determine later disputes and define the rights and duties of healthcare professionals, including doctors, and patients in areas not covered by statutes. The law of negligence imposes a duty of care not to injure the patient unreasonably. This includes making a diagnosis, giving advice, and undertaking the treatment of a patient. Common law governs questions of compensation for medical accidents or negligence but also covers several other vital matters. It is beyond the scope of this chapter to explore the wider underpinning matters of medical ethics, and readers are encouraged to read more extensively.

Why is the law of medical negligence important?

There are several reasons why the law relating to medical negligence is so important.
- It is often regarded as the greatest incentive to develop and maintain patient safety.
- Adverse events that cause patient harm can lead to massive compensation claims that have to be paid by the healthcare provider.

- High-profile court cases can undermine confidence in the healthcare provider, including both individual healthcare workers and the organizations within which they work.
- The trigger for patients who are negligently harmed to pursue a claim through the courts for compensation may result from an initial failure on the part of the provider of care, including the healthcare professional, to offer an adequate explanation or apology.
- Not every negligently harmed patient sues; indeed, the vast majority do not sue.
- An action for perceived negligence may succeed because of a failure to document the process of care adequately and clearly.

The standard of care and negligence

Any person can be considered to be negligent if they have failed to act reasonably by reference to the standards of the hypothetical ordinary reasonable person – the so-called 'man on the Clapham omnibus'. The legal test for medical (or 'clinical') negligence was set out in the case of *Bolam v Friern Hospital Management Committee* (Box 9.1). In deciding the level of competence there may be one or more perfectly acceptable standards.

The legal process of establishing negligence

There are two stages to this process of law.
1 First, there must be an assessment by the court of how, in the circumstances, the defendant ought to have behaved – what standard of care should the doctor have exercised? This enquiry requires a judgment to be made, and expert opinion is usually considered.
2 Then there must be a decision about whether on the facts of the case (as determined from the evidence) the defendant's conduct fell below the appropriate standard. This latter element is a question of fact rather than law.

Box 9.1 **The Bolam Test**

A doctor is not guilty of negligence if he has acted in accordance with a practice accepted as proper by a responsible body of medical men skilled in the particular art … Putting it the other way round, a doctor is not negligent, if he is acting in accordance with such a practice, merely because there is a body of opinion that takes a contrary view. Mr Justice McNair in the Bolam case [1957] 2 All ER 118

The courts apply a number of general principles in reaching their judgment about what standard of care ought to be applied. In broad terms, the courts undertake a crude cost–benefit analysis in which the magnitude of the risk of harm (how likely was it to occur; how serious was the potential harm?) is weighed against the burden of avoiding the risk and the potential benefits to the patient of running the risk (Box 9.2, Fig. 9.1).

- The standard of care expected of the reasonable professional is objective. It does not take account of the individual attributes of the particular defendant, such as inexperience. The inexperienced professional can avoid liability by having his or her work checked by a more senior colleague. It is also not possible to argue that an adequate service has been provided most of the time and that a practitioner should be excused when occasionally falling below an acceptable standard. If a patient is harmed as a result of a failure to exercise reasonable care, the fact that the rest of the patient's care was exemplary provides no defence.
- A defendant is liable only for foreseeable harm; risks that could not have been foreseen at the time of the adverse event are not taken into account. It is the defendant's obligation to exercise reasonable care, not take absolute care, and what is reasonable varies with the circumstances. In some circumstances it may be reasonable to ig-nore a small foreseeable risk, for example where the potential benefits are great. So the defendant's purpose for acting in a particular way will be taken into account. For example, an attempt at saving a limb will justify the taking of greater risk than in routine care.
- Negligence takes account of the practicability of taking precautions against the risk. If only comparatively small improvements in safety can be achieved by the expenditure of a large amount of resource, it may be reasonable not to undertake precautions. This is a measure of the objective reasonableness of the defendant's conduct. It does not mean that a defendant's lack of resources can justify a failure to take precautions that would otherwise be re-garded as reasonably required.

Expert evidence and negligence

Both defendant and claimant may produce conflicting expert evidence construed as from responsible bodies of professional opinion. A potentially justifiable claim may fail because of this conflict of opinion. It is essential that expert evidence must stand up to logical analysis. In particular in cases involving, as they so often do, the weighing of risks against benefits, the judge will need to be satisfied that, in forming their views, the experts have directed their minds to the question of comparative risks and benefits and have reached a defensible conclusion on the matter (see *Bolitho v City and Hackney Health Authority* (1997)). It is anticipated that only rarely will professional opinion be incapable of withstanding logical analysis.

Adverse events and litigation

The relationship between medical mishap and litigation is an unknown. It is estimated that 850 000 adverse events (about 10% of all hospitalizations) occur each year in National Health Service (NHS) hospitals in England, of which half are avoidable. The number of avoidable adverse events caused by negligence is not known. In one large US study an estimated 4% of hospitalized patients suffered an adverse event, of which one quarter (or 1%) suffered injury of varying degree as a result of negligence. Applying that figure to England one might expect over 85 000 new negligent adverse events a year. This contrasts with around 6000 new claims per year being dealt with by the NHS Litigation Authority, of which about 60% may be unsuccessful (Box 9.3).

The argument from a policy perspective for medical litigation is that it acts as a deterrent for wrongful conduct of the defendant by imposing liability. However, this relationship is tenuous, not least

---

Box 9.2 Magnitude of the risk of harm

The courts consider two factors:
1 the likely incidence of harm;
2 the probable severity of any harm that may occur.
The consequence is that if the risk of injury occurring is very small, it may be reasonable simply to ignore the risk, and take no precautions against it; on the other hand, if the damage, should it materialize, be severe, it may be negligent to ignore even a small risk.

Box 9.3 Reasons for not proceeding to litigation by patients who have suffered an adverse event

- They may not know about the process or realize that they are eligible.
- People may be more accepting of more minor harm if corrective action is taken, an explanation given and apology offered.
- Making a claim is potentially demanding in time, emotion and cost, and individuals may be reluctant to travel this path.
- Patients may be more accepting of degrees of error in a service that is free, or feel future access may be thwarted should they create a fuss.

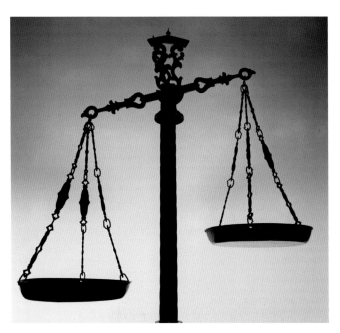

Figure 9.1 The legal balance of risk vs benefit. (Image courtesy of Getty Images.)

Table 9.1 Claims for clinical and nonclinical negligence against the National Health Service for the period 2003–2006, and corresponding amounts paid out (damages and legal costs combined)

Year	Clinical negligence claims	Cost (£ million)	Nonclinical negligence claims	Cost (£ million)
2003–04	6251	422.5	3819	10.1
2004–05	5609	502.9	3766	25.1
2005–06	5697	560.3	3497	31.3

because most professionals carry some form of medical indemnity or are covered as a result of employment within the NHS. The burden of liability does not fall directly on the defendant apart from potential damage to reputation. Neither the insurers nor the NHS have clear strategies in place for linking the compensation process back to individuals (Box 9.4).

Defensive medicine

A perceived consequence of the threat of medical litigation is defensive medicine. This arises when practitioners undertake investigations and procedures that are not medically justified for the patient's benefit but are pursued to protect the doctor from a claim for negligence. The most commonly cited examples are unnecessary diagnostic tests such as X-rays and unnecessary Caesarean sections. However, if this situation is true, and given the increased risks associated with invasive tasks or procedures, the doctor may be at increased risk of being successfully sued for negligence. It is more likely that defensive medicine represents a more careful or conservative approach to patient management at the expense of cost efficiency and cost benefits.

The important element from a legal perspective is that the judgement involved in determining the choice of investigation and treatment is an objective one in exercising reasonable standards or professional conduct. Defensive practice may be a double-edged sword in either changing good practice into bad practice (too many unjustifiable tests) or deterring poor practice by encouraging stricter adherence to good practice guidelines.

Improving patient safety by responding to litigation

The function of the legal process is to attribute legal responsibility for the consequences of one or more adverse events. It does not identify root causes or systemic failures in services. Also, not all possible claims proceed through a public court process, and only those cases that cause the greatest damage or loss are likely to proceed through litigation. Very occasionally there may be a specific response by the NHS to specific incidents, such as the changes introduced following the scandal of organ retention at Alder Hey hospital.

It is difficult to prove that a healthcare organization is at fault, particularly where the practice at fault is commonly adopted throughout the NHS. For example, it may be common practice to leave the most junior and therefore inexperienced staff on the frontline of healthcare delivery, partly through lack of resources and partly as a means of giving hands-on training. It would be difficult for a judge to condemn as negligent a practice widely adopted in the NHS, even if this is recognized as increasing the risk of harm to patients, because to address it would require major financial and political investment. Under these circumstances judges find it easier to conclude that the individual practitioner at the end of the chain of responsibility was negligent, and then hold the organization vicariously liable for that individual's negligent mistake.

Extent of litigation and costs in the NHS

Table 9.1 summarizes the numbers of claims for clinical and nonclinical negligence received by the NHS Litigation Authority (NHSLA) in the three years from 2003 to 2006. The costs given include both damages paid to patients and the legal costs borne by the NHS. Birth-related claims account for 20% of claims but 60% of the financial payout.

At 31 March 2006 the NHSLA estimated that its total liabilities (the theoretical cost of paying all outstanding claims immediately, including those relating to incidents that have occurred but have not yet been reported to) were £8.2 billion for clinical claims and £0.14 billion for nonclinical claims.

An analysis of all clinical claims handled by the NHSLA between 1 April 1996 and 31 March 2006 shows that 38% were abandoned by the claimant, 43% settled out of court, 4% settled in court and 15% remain outstanding.

Further reading

Brazier M. *Medicine, Patients and the Law*, 3rd edn. Penguin Books, London, 2003.

Donaldson, L. *Making Amends: A Consultation Paper Setting out Proposals for Reforming the Approach to Clinical Negligence in the NHS*. The Stationery Office, London, 2003.

Jones M. *Medical Negligence*, 3rd edn. Sweet & Maxwell, London, 2003.

Kennedy I, Grubb A. *Medical Law*, 3rd edn. Butterworths, London, 2000.

Mason JK, Laurie GT. *Mason & McCall Smith's Law and Medical Ethics*, 7th edn. Oxford University Press, Oxford, 2006.

National Health Service Litigation Authority. Factsheets 2 and 3, available from the NHSLA website (www.nhsla.com).

Rosenthal MM, Sutcliffe KM (eds). *Medical Error: What Do We Know? What Do We Do?* Jossey-Bass, San Francisco, 2002.

Walshe K, Boaden R (eds) *Patient Safety: Research into Practice*. Open University Press, Maidenhead, 2006, Chapter 6.

CHAPTER 10

The Healthcare Policy Context

Robert L Phillips

OVERVIEW

- Approaches to improving patient safety have been slow to develop
- There is now a global programme for the development of patient safety policy
- Major policy initiatives include the implementation of incident reporting systems and computerization of healthcare processes
- Improving quality may provide the most effective long-term approach to improving patient safety

Institute of Medicine's hugely influential report *To Err is Human: Building a Safer Health System*, which through its highly successful marketing approach direct to the US media and public made such an impact. There has subsequently been an increasing impetus to develop patient safety initiatives in many countries of the world, especially the USA, UK, Australia and Germany. This train of movement in patient safety has resulted in a global programme of policy development, culminating in the formation of the World Health Organization's World Alliance for Patient Safety (Figs 10.1 and 10.2).

Over the last two decades, there has been an increasing awareness and acceptance of the extent, and subsequent cost, of the actual harm that patients can suffer during healthcare. This has jolted all healthcare providers into action. The result has been an increasing number of policies and strategies that have been designed to ensure patient safety.

Overall approaches to improve quality in healthcare can also improve patient safety. These approaches include setting, delivering and monitoring standards. For example, clear standards of delivery, such as guidelines, and professional regulation can improve patient safety.

The landmark Harvard study suggested that deaths equivalent to one jumbo-jet crash per day were occurring as a direct result of preventable harm in US hospitals. However, it was almost a decade after publication of this study that the world's interest in medical errors was really ignited. The catalyst was the launch in 2000 of the

LONDON DECLARATION
Patients for Patient Safety

WHO World Alliance for Patient Safety

We, Patients for Patient Safety, pledge to help create a world in which health care errors harm fewer people. We, gathered in London from 27-30 November 2005 to join together in partnership in an effort to reduce the massive burden of avoidable harm in health care. Risk and uncertainty are constant companions. So we come together in dialogue, participating in care with providers. We unite our strength as advocates for care with less harm in the developing as well as the developed world.

We are committed to spreading the word from person to person, town to town, country to country. There is a right to safe health care and we will not let the current culture of error and denial continue. We call for honesty, openness and transparency. We will make the reduction of health-care errors a basic human right that protects human life around the world.

We, Patients for Patient Safety, will be the voice of all patients, but especially of those who are now unheard. Together, as partners, we will collaborate in:

- Devising and promoting programmes for patient safety and patient empowerment.
- Developing and driving a constructive dialogue with all partners concerned with patient safety.
- Establishing systems for reporting and dealing with health-care harm on a worldwide basis.
- Defining best practices that deal with health-care harm of all kinds and promote those practices throughout the world.

In honor of those who have died, those who have been left disabled and our loved ones today, we will strive for excellence, so that all people receiving health care are as safe as possible, as soon as possible. This is our pledge of partnership.

January 17, 2006

Figure 10.2 London declaration by Patients for Patient Safety (www.who.int/entity/patientsafety/information_centre/Final_London_Declaration_Feb06.pdf).

World Health Organization

| | 中文 | English | Français | Русский | Español |

Home
About WHO
Countries
Health topics
Publications
Research tools
WHO sites
Patient safety
Alliance launch
Global challenge
Patients for patient safety
Taxonomy
Research

Patient safety

Events | Links | Contact us

WHO > WHO sites

Patient safety

In October 2004, WHO launched the World Alliance for Patient Safety in response to a World Health Assembly Resolution (2002) urging WHO and Member States to pay the closest possible attention to the problem of patient safety. The Alliance raises awareness and political commitment to improve the safety of care and facilitates the development of patient safety policy and practice in all WHO Member States. Each year, the Alliance delivers a number of programmes covering systemic and technical aspects to improve patient safety around the world.

Technical experts worldwide
This is a restricted access area for the Alliance technical experts.
Access here

PATIENT SAFETY NEWS

China
October 2006
China Focuses on Improving Drug Safety
More information

South Africa
October 2006
The Council for Health Service Accreditation of Southern Africa
More information [pdf]

Figure 10.1 The World Health Organization's World Alliance for Patient Safety represents an important international advance.

The development of the patient safety movement

The USA was the first to develop a patient safety movement, but its development has been fragmentary. The National Patient Safety Foundation (NPSF) was established in 1996 as the first international organization dedicated to patient safety. This non-profit-making and independent organization has continued to lead in building a knowledge base, in creating forums to share knowledge, and in facilitating improvement programmes. At the same time, a variety of stakeholders established their own initiatives: the Joint Commission on Accreditation of Health Care Organizations (JCAHO) was established; the healthcare provider Veterans Administration developed the National Center for Patient Safety (NCPS); and business leaders who purchase health insurance convened the Leapfrog Group. Moreover, the US government established the National Quality Forum (NQF) in an attempt to bring together the many organizations involved in healthcare (Box 10.1).

In the UK, the impetus to develop patient safety was the report by the Chief Medical Officer (CMO) entitled *An Organisation With A Memory*. This report was quickly followed by *Building a Safer NHS for Patients*, which operationalized the strategy. Subsequently, the National Patient Safety Agency (NPSA) was established. The NPSA has established the National Reporting and Learning System (NRLS) and an active development and educational programme for both primary and secondary care (Fig. 10.3).

> **Box 10.1 Rules for healthcare redesign**
>
> - Care based on continuous healing relationships
> - Customization based on patient needs and values
> - The patient as the source of control
> - Shared knowledge and the free flow of information
> - Evidence-based decision-making
> - Safety as a system priority
> - The need for transparency
> - Anticipation of needs
> - Continuous decrease in waste
> - Cooperation among clinicians
>
> (From Committee on Quality of Health Care in America, 2001.)

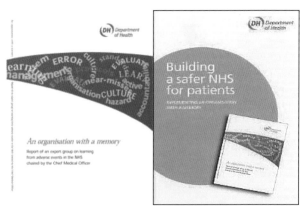

Figure 10.3 The Department of Health's strategic policy documents have proved extremely influential.

> **Box 10.2 Six key areas of activity for the WHO's World Alliance for Patient Safety Programme**
>
> 1 Formulation of a Global Patient Safety Challenge
> 2 Patient and consumer involvement
> 3 Developing a patient safety taxonomy
> 4 Research in the field of patient safety
> 5 Solutions to reduce the risk of healthcare and improve its safety
> 6 Reporting and learning to improve patient safety

A framework for understanding present initiatives in patient safety

The World Alliance for Patient Safety was launched by the World Health Organization (WHO) in October 2004 with the aim of realizing the maxim 'First do no harm' by cutting the number of iatrogenic illnesses, injuries and deaths suffered by patients. The Alliance has developed six key areas of work, an appreciation of which allows individual countries better to appreciate their progress towards patient safety (Box 10.2).

Using this framework, it is clear that some countries, such as the USA, UK and Australia, have accomplished the recognition phase and are well on their way to characterizing the contexts in which errors are most likely to occur and their underlying causes, but progress in identifying evidence-based approaches to prevent adverse events and then to ensure that these are implemented and sustained has been less developed. The situation in many transition and economically developing countries, however, remains very much upstream of this, reflecting the enormity of the challenge that lies ahead.

Latest trends in patient safety policy

Error reporting

The UK is far ahead of the USA in implementing error reporting, having created the National Reporting and Learning System (NRLS). Australia has one of the most mature and well-studied systems for reporting errors, emphasizing ease of reporting, classifying errors and contributing factors against a standardized terminology as a report is made, and generating more immediate feedback to reporters. The Australian system offers many lessons in improving reporting and the effectiveness of reporting systems for improving safety. The NRLS and Australian Incident Monitoring System are already confidential and anonymous. The US Patient Safety and Quality Improvement Act of 2005 will establish a confidential reporting structure in which healthcare professionals can voluntarily report on errors to designated patient safety organizations. This legislation will help remove some barriers to implementing reporting of patient safety incidents.

After implementation there are still practical barriers to a national reporting system. One acute NHS trust's adverse incident reporting system already reports receiving an average of 22 reports per day. If this is a typical volume across trusts, it runs the risk of sustaining criticism of such systems – the incapacity to analyse reports adequately and produce information that can prevent similar adverse events for future patients. Such a system could attract reports of 0.5 to 5 million near misses annually in the USA, and the report review costs per case would be very large. Achieving the real value of reporting systems will require purposeful capacity to store, retrieve, analyse and systematically learn from huge volumes of incident reports. Most existing reporting systems have struggled with this capacity, and there has been insufficient investment in studying it.

Computerization of practice

The UK National Programme for Information Technology aims to connect 30 000 general practitioners and 300 hospitals and give patients access to their personal health records. This effort is as important for standardizing platforms of health information and the promise of interconnectivity of information as it is for widely distributing the technology. In the USA, there is considerable pressure on hospitals to institute computer physician order entry systems. Lack of standards and implementation support has made this effort fitful. There is some evidence that general practice in the USA is seeing increased computerization; however, lack of any financial support for purchasing IT systems, for implementing them, for transferring information from paper charts or for associated breaks in practice makes this change patchy at best. The USA also currently lacks standards for health IT systems, which are essential to ensure smooth data transfer between healthcare providers. The UK Care Record Development Board should help the UK overcome similar challenges.

Once there is sufficient computerization of practice, and standards supporting secure connectivity are in place, the goal of using informatics to improve quality and safety will still be only partly realized. Surgeries and trusts will need to be able to query patient and practice data routinely and turn it into information about the delivery of high-quality, safe care. Such studies can also drive the improvement of decision support tools within practice IT systems by tailoring them to the epidemiology and demographics that determine the predictive disease models of each practice. Queries can also generate feedback to physicians and practices, and permit peer comparisons that motivate change.

Safety culture

Moving healthcare organizations to achieve shared beliefs, norms and values related to quality and safety is the ultimate goal of achieving a culture of safety. The UK prominently leads this effort, and there are pockets of focused activity in the USA, particularly in acute care and hospital settings. Tools that can reliably measure safety culture are still developing, but the NPSA already has one instrument that it plans to use across the NHS. Sustaining the patient safety movement will depend on being able to make and measure lasting culture changes within practices and healthcare systems (Box 10.3). See also Boxes 10.4–10.6.

Is patient safety losing steam or merely changing focus?

Safety is but one aspect of high-quality healthcare; however, it has been a very important stimulus for improving healthcare quality. In the USA, there has been a precipitous decline in funding for pa-

Box 10.3 **The National Patient Safety Agency's 'Seven steps to patient safety for primary care'**

Step 1: Build a safety culture – create a culture that is open and fair.
Step 2: Lead and support your staff – establish a clear and strong focus on patient safety throughout your organization.
Step 3: Integrate your risk management activity – develop systems and processes to manage your risks and identify and assess things that could go wrong.
Step 4: Promote reporting – ensure your staff can easily report incidents locally and nationally.
Step 5: Involve and communicate with patients and the public – develop ways to communicate openly with and listen to patients.
Step 6: Learn and share safety lessons – encourage staff to use root cause analysis and significant event auditing to learn how and why incidents happen.
Step 7: Implement solutions to prevent harm – embed lessons through changes to practice, processes or systems.

Box 10.4 **NPSA definition of patient safety incidents**

Any unintended or unexpected incident which could have or did lead to harm of one or more patients receiving NHS-funded care

Box 10.5 **Key areas for patient safety improvement**

• A unified system for reporting and analysis when things go wrong
• A more open culture in which errors or service failures can be reported and discussed
• Mechanisms for ensuring that, where lessons are identified, the necessary changes are put into practice
• A wider appreciation of the value of the system approach in preventing, analysing and learning from errors
(After Department of Health, 2000.)

Box 10.6 **Quality approaches that can improve patient safety**

• **Setting clear standards of delivery:**
  National guidelines, e.g. National Institute for Clinical Excellence (NICE)
  Service delivery standards, e.g. National Service Frameworks (NSF)
• **Dependable delivery of care**
  Clinical governance procedures, including audit
  Lifelong learning
  Professional regulation
• **Monitoring standards**
  Accreditation bodies
• User involvement, e.g. National Patient and User Survey

tient safety research, but it has never amounted to more than 0.2% of the funding allocated to the National Institutes of Health. The UK has instituted a contract for general practice that promotes specific measures of quality that, if met, promise increased income. Although this is not specifically tailored to improve safety, the commitment of new resources to improved quality may promote new systems and team functions, and a culture change that will also support safety. This real 'pay for performance' is accompanied by government support for computerization and serious efforts to measure elements of safe culture quantitatively and qualitatively. This approach is more comprehensive than the approach in the USA, which, while not finalized, has lacked the evidence-based approach and commitment of new resources.

Advancing quality is a broader strategy, more positive in its focus, and probably better for marshalling resources and passion than safety in the long run. Healthcare will always be complex and uncertain, and carry a real risk of harming patients. A shift to quality as the dominant focus may be for the best, but improving safety should be retained as a specific component of this effort.

Further reading

Committee on Quality of Health Care in America. *Crossing the Quality Chasm: a New Health System for the 21st Century.* National Academy Press, Washington DC, 2001.

Department of Health. *An Organisation with Memory. Report of an Expert Group on Learning from Adverse Events in the NHS.* The Stationery Office, London 2000 (http://www.npsa.nhs.uk/site/media/documents/345_org.pdf).

Kohn LT, Corrigan JM, Donaldson MS (eds). *To Err Is Human: Building a Safer Health System.* The National Academies Press, Washington DC, 2000.

National Patient Safety Agency. *Introduction to Patient Safety e-learning* (http://www.npsa.nhs.uk/health/resources/ipsel).

National Patient Safety Agency. *Seven Steps to Patient Safety in Primary Care* (http://www.npsa.nhs.uk/web/display?contentId=2664).

Walshe K, Boaden R (eds). *Patient Safety: Research into Practice.* Open University Press, Maidenhead, 2005.

CHAPTER 11

The Impact on Patients and Healthcare Professionals

Amanda Howe, Peter Walsh

OVERVIEW

- Both patients and healthcare staff suffer from a patient safety incident
- Patients and carers often make a complaint or begin litigation if they have not been given an initial explanation about a patient safety incident
- Most healthcare professionals have been educated to believe in perfection
- Support services are available to healthcare professionals who are suffering from the aftermath of a complaint or litigation

Box 11.1 **What matters most to patients when something goes wrong**

- 34% wanted an explanation/apology for what went wrong.
- 23% wanted an inquiry into causes.
- 17% want support in coping with the result.
- 11% seek financial compensation.
- 7% seek disciplinary action on the professionals involved.

(After Department of Health report *Making Amends* (2003).)

Box 11.2 **Dealing with complaints**

- Do not ignore.
- Act quickly and speak to the patient making the complaint.
- Acknowledge how the complainant feels about the situation.
- Establish what the complainant is hoping for in complaining.
- It is okay to say sorry.
- You do not have to admit that you are at fault and guilty.

Box 11.3 **Obstacles that patients have to overcome before a complaint is made**

- Fear of care being removed
- Fear of being stigmatized as a 'complainer' and subsequent prejudice to future care they may receive
- Fear of an unknown process
- Fear of being regarded as 'uncharitable' and ungrateful of receiving healthcare

If problems arise with patient safety, both patients and healthcare staff suffer. For patients, there is the impact of the problem itself, usually coupled with negative emotions (such as anger, confusion or disappointment), the need to deal with the reactions of others, and a variety of lost opportunities, such as career or financial, which are a consequence of the problem. For staff, there is guilt at letting themselves and their patients down, and sometimes there is the potential loss of career and earnings, especially if the problem harms their reputation in the longer term.

Effect on patients of threats to patient safety

In spite of alarmist media headlines about harm inflicted during medical care, doctors are the most trusted of all professions. It invariably comes as a shock to patients and their carers when something goes wrong during their care. Most people are remarkably understanding despite the personal trauma caused by any physical harm. They also have to cope with the feeling of having been let down by the people in whom they place great trust.

Why make a complaint or begin litigation?

People are often motivated to seek disciplinary action or compensation only when they perceive that there has been an initial denial or an attempt at cover-up. Patients have a right to expect openness and honesty, but the only statutory right afforded in the UK to patients who have been affected by a medical error is to invoke the NHS complaints procedure or to take legal action. Sometimes these actions are an attempt to try and get to the truth and ensure lessons are learned that may help others. However, patients and family members often need to obtain compensation to help cope with the implications of injuries caused through negligence, and it is a legitimate right to seek it. A clinical negligence action should not necessarily be seen as a personal attack on an individual professional but as the only method to obtain compensation from the healthcare system to which the professional belongs (Boxes 11.1–11.3).

Effect on doctors of patient safety initiatives and complaints

All doctors are constantly reminded to improve patient safety through a variety of methods, from guidelines to reminders, but only when things go wrong, or when there is a 'near miss', do doctors really make an effort to change their practice. Thus complaints can be useful in ensuring that lessons are learned, and other patients do not run similar risks in the future.

However, problems can be deeply distressing to the doctor – 'the second victim'. When a doctor realizes an error has occurred, he or she usually goes through a range of emotions, such as shock, distress, denial, anger, grief and regret. These powerful emotions can significantly impair the personal and professional functioning of the doctor.

Many doctors have been taught in an environment that expects perfection and is unforgiving of error. This is compounded by the frequent pre-existing personality trait of being a natural worrier. An initial reaction to any error is usually that of personal failure. Litigation is often regarded as being unjustified, and attempts at settling a claim are felt to be an admission of guilt. This feeling of guilt is reinforced with anger. Subsequently, the doctor may begin to become totally consumed with concern and begin to experience sleeplessness, loss of appetite, indecisiveness and thoughts that constantly return to the incident. In severe cases, panic attacks and depression can occur. Occasionally, doctors have committed suicide.

Learning from safety incidents

Services and patients often do not distinguish between the issues of accountability and learning. Yet, often, the greatest wish of patients and carers is for the incident to be recognized, its root causes identified, and remedies put in place so that the likelihood of the problem being replicated is reduced. Some of the thematic work carried out by the National Patient Safety Agency with patients and carers, for example on infusion devices, anticoagulants, dispensing errors, blood transfusions, gynaecological services and hospital-acquired infections, suggests that patients and carers welcome the opportunity to contribute to this work by helping to define the factors that shape and cause patient safety incidents. It also helps them emotionally because there is some satisfaction in knowing that a patient safety incident that harmed them or their loved ones can contribute to patient safety in the future.

Support for staff harmed by errors

Most doctors will feel devastated by a complaint, whether or not they feel personally at fault, and will experience stress and a loss of confidence while these emotional reactions are taking place. The role of others in support and taking shared responsibility therefore becomes crucial (Box 11.4).

A doctor may be falsely accused, or wholly blamed for something that is only partly his or her fault. The health system and the law usually accuse an individual, although the patient safety literature indicates that most errors arise from systems failures. This can have further adverse effects because others involved are often delighted to absent themselves, while the individual focuses on the unfairness of the situation rather than on their own needs and responsibilities. To avoid this, professionals need to be prepared by their training to accept and work constructively on their response to complaints, usually by being encouraged to exercise emotional insight and in-

Box 11.4 **Assisting staff who have had a complaint made against them**

- Prompt response to all stages of the process
- Offer of supportive counselling
- Support from managers
- Regular feedback on progress of a case
- Training in effective handling of complaints

tellectual objectivity. Another aspect is that the individual doctor becomes 'stuck' in their distress and guilt, and develops a depressive reaction, which can cause further problems. A final aspect is that they will be unable to engage with the patients and their families, who will generally need an honest explanation and apology (if justified) to be able to come to terms with their own distress and anger.

In order to get the best rather than the worst out of these distressing situations, doctors need role models that can show them how to handle difficult situations well. They need a person who is available to them for nonjudgemental support and who can also understand the full picture, especially the formal complaint and litigation process. An important role of the healthcare organization is to respond quickly to all stages of the process of any complaint and to keep the doctor informed of the complaint's progress. It is particularly useful to have a named person who can monitor the progress of both the complaint and the doctor's approach to coping with the complaint.

BMA Counselling Service: **provides doctors and their families with 24-hour telephone counselling by qualified counsellors. Tel. 0845 920 0169.**

Requirements for education and training: developing a patient safety curriculum

Effectively responding to adverse events and complaints requires a range of skills. Communication skills are essential when things do go wrong, and although there are many general skills, such as active listening, there are more specific skills, such as saying sorry. However, skills training has to be supplemented by methods that increase awareness of the emotional reaction that the patient is going through and the possible reasons for the actions of the patient. Involvement of knowledgeable patient organizations such as Action against Medical Accidents (AvMA) is also an important ingredient in educating doctors because they can provide 'expert patients' who can clearly describe their reactions to medical errors. All doctors also need to develop an understanding of their own emotional reactions to adverse events and complaints, and how these emotions can interfere with their communication with patients.

The culture of the healthcare organization has become increasingly important in understanding how patient safety is developed and maintained in a healthcare organization. There are significant parallels between the culture of medical education and the safety culture of an organization. The relationship between the teacher and learner is fundamental in all education, but in medicine there is often a culture dominated by 'blame and shame'. Learners do not disclose lack of confidence or competence when facing a situation, yet both are common causes of major threats to patient safety. A hierarchical and competitive atmosphere is often present, and teaching frequently still occurs by humiliation of the learner. These pose important challenges to all medical educators.

Students can learn by observing role models, especially when participating in the investigation of adverse events, such as root cause analyses. Important to learning is openness about both the facts of the particular case and the emotional reaction experienced by those involved. The development of role models in doctors who have

---

Box 11.5 **The culture of medical education**

- Competitiveness
- 'Shame and blame'
- Humiliation by tutors
- Lack of role models

Box 11.6 **Methods for education and training in effective communication after a medical error or complaint**

- Simulated patients on which to practise communication skills
- Observing complaints officers at work
- Live encounters with patients and patient advocates to increase awareness of the patient perspective
- Live encounters with doctors who have had complaints so as to talk about the emotional aspects and how they coped both personally and professionally

---

a responsibility for training is essential, but it is also necessary for the wider organization to have these characteristics, otherwise the learner will not be able transfer their learning (Box 11.5).

A specific patient safety curriculum may be proposed, but patient safety is a wide concept, and there are many instances of specific knowledge or skills, such as safe prescribing, that need to be considered. However, these are often part of existing programmes of instruction (Box 11.6).

Further reading

Walshe K, Boaden R (eds). *Patient Safety: Research into Practice.* Open University Press, Maidenhead, 2005.

Further resources

Support for patients and carers
Action against Medical Accidents (http://www.avma.org.uk/index.asp). Helpline: 0845 123 23 52.

Support for doctors in the UK
Association of Anaesthetists' Sick Doctor Scheme: Advice for anaesthetists. Tel. 020 7631 1650.

BMA Counselling Service: provides doctors and their families with 24-hour telephone counselling by qualified counsellors. Tel. 0845 920 0169.

British International Doctors' Association: where cultural or linguistic differences may be a contributing factor, doctors can access the health counselling panel. Tel. 0161 456 7828 (email: oda@doctors.org.uk).

Royal College of Obstetricians and Gynaecologists: provides mentoring support for Members and Fellows in difficulties. Tel. 020 7772 6369 (www.rcog.org.uk).

Royal College of Surgeons Confidential Support and Advice Service (CSAS): helpline providing confidential surgeon-to-surgeon help. Tel. 0800 107 1916 (www.rcseng.ac.uk/support/csas).

CHAPTER 12

Future Directions

Aziz Sheikh, Maureen Baker, Richard Thomson

OVERVIEW

- Patient safety is still a major concern for all healthcare providers
- The main barrier to improving patient safety is organizational blocks to implementation
- There is little evidence base to demonstrate the effectiveness of patient safety interventions
- Further research is required to influence policy and practice

---

Patient safety remains a major concern for all healthcare providers. There are still regular headlines in the press that shock everyone who provides, and also receives, healthcare. These patient safety incidents are only the tip of the iceberg, and there are numerous events, actual and potential, that pose threats to patient safety.

What has been achieved so far in patient safety

Recently, Leape and Berwick looked back over the five years in US healthcare since the publication in 2000 of *To Err is Human: Building a Safer Health System*. They noted that there have been important changes, with improvement in patient safety in a small number of practices, such as reduction in the accidental injection of potassium chloride, but that overall there has been little major improvement (Box 12.1).

Box 12.1 **Achievements in patient safety so far**

- Increased awareness of healthcare organizations, care givers and patients of the importance and extent of threats to patient safety.
- Enlistment of a range of stakeholders to advance patient safety, including the development of government organizations, such as the National Patient Safety Foundation (NPSF) and the National Patient Safety Agency (NPSA), professional associations and patient groups.
- Changing practices, such as the introduction of methods to reduce the chances of wrong-site surgery.

(After Leape & Berwick, 2005.)

Barriers to progress in patient safety

A large range of policies and procedures have been developed to improve safety. The barrier does not appear to be lack of ideas but is due to problems with their implementation to produce lasting change in practice. It is important to recognize that all healthcare is complex, and that there is no simple solution, but a major barrier appears to be the culture of healthcare. Healthcare is often fragmented across several care-givers, and everyone has to accept that they have an individual responsibility for patient safety, and that they also have to be willing to work with the various professional groups that are usually required for effective healthcare (Boxes 12.2 and 12.3).

Future directions to improve patient safety

A lot can be learnt from progress in other safety critical industries, such as nuclear power, petrochemicals and aerospace. An important and overarching concept is a positive approach to patient safety. This requires both an individual and a collective mindset

---

Box 12.2 **Complexity and patient safety**

- Problems presented to healthcare providers are often complex.
- Effective healthcare is complex, requiring a wide range of interventions and professionals.
- Healthcare organizations are complex systems, and organizational change is difficult.
- Patient safety interventions are complex, and have often been developed in non-healthcare contexts.

Box 12.3 **Cultural barriers in healthcare**

- Scepticism about proposed changes to improve patient safety
- Individual autonomy with lack of willingness to work collaboratively
- High individual responsibility for actions with self-blame for errors
- Fear of complaints and litigation that leads to lack of willingness to admit and discuss errors
- Hierarchical structure that blames individuals instead of systems

---

of 'How can I ensure that this activity is the safest possible for the patient?' whenever any action is contemplated. This proactive approach requires increased vigilance; it is not an optional extra but an integral part of good clinical practice. A negative attitude to safety regards an error as something that is not inevitable but can be prevented by a process in which errors are actively identified. However, it may be that such an approach can actually worsen safety. The logic is that this process can produce an image of an unsafe organization, and this destroys the collective mental image of safe procedures that the workers within the organization have developed (Box 12.4).

Leadership

Countries in which there has been significant progress towards enhancing patient safety share the characteristics of being mature democracies in which clear leadership has been displayed by people in positions of power within healthcare systems. For example, in England and Wales the challenge of transforming the safety record of the NHS has been led by the Chief Medical Officer in England, who shortly after the launch of the Institute of Medicine's report *To Err is Human: Building a Safer Health System* published the Department of Health's extremely influential plan to create *An Organisation with a Memory*. There is a clear need for leadership at the highest possible level if the safety agenda is to generate the support it warrants. In addition, it is crucial that the importance of local leadership is not overlooked, for example, at the level of hospitals and clinical teams. There is advice in *Seven Steps to Patient Safety*, the National Patient Safety Agency's guide, on leading and supporting staff as a focus on patient safety is being embedded in a healthcare organization's culture.

Conceptual clarity

Although there has been considerable advance in thinking about the nature of clinical risk, medical errors and patient safety, there is still the need for greater clarity of the strengths and limitations of these various concepts, and the interrelationship and boundaries between them. For example, whilst patient safety as a concept has considerable advantages in that it is a nonpejorative term, it has the disadvantage of being less clearly defined than more limited concepts such as adverse events – indeed, the boundaries of patient safety and quality are difficult to characterize, and what is considered as sitting within the domain of safety is still open to debate. For example, is failure to implement evidence-based guidance a safety or quality of care issue? For these reasons, quantitative epidemiological studies have focused largely on the study of error or adverse event rates, both of which are potentially measurable but are indirect measures of safety.

An attempt at an international glossary of key terms will be fundamental to the long-term progress of the discipline. This will also be an essential prerequisite to the World Alliance for Patient Safety's attempt to develop a unified, theoretically informed taxonomy of patient safety.

Coherent national policies

The move to prioritize patient safety by healthcare systems is important, but there still remains a great deal of scepticism on the part of clinicians, who feel that by sharing highly sensitive information they may still be subject to the threat and penalties historically associated with errors, in particular litigation, disciplinary procedures and adverse publicity. Progress in this respect will need far more enlightened policies, for example the promotion of an 'open and fair' culture, where clinicians are actively encouraged to report errors for the purpose of learning and where action that improves safety and feedback on this is seen to happen as a result of such reporting.

Research must focus on developing and evaluating the effectiveness of interventions

The increasing body of work on the epidemiology of patient safety incidents suggests broadly similar pictures in the developed healthcare systems – that such incidents are common in secondary care and responsible for considerable disease burden. There is thus perhaps relatively little to be gained internationally by further purely descriptive work studying the burden posed by errors in secondary care, unless this work is undertaken as a catalyst for national action or is being undertaken in parts of the world with very different healthcare systems from those already studied. The epidemiology of errors in primary care remains poorly characterized, and there is some merit in the argument that a large national study is still warranted. That said, the existing databases of errors and adverse events will offer considerable insight, particularly if there are mechanisms to allow effective and efficient sharing of information between systems internationally. However, this may prove problematic for a number of reasons including different taxonomies of patient safety incidents, methods of collecting data (e.g. anonymous vs open; mandatory vs voluntary) and analysis (e.g. qualitative vs quantitative).

There is now a wealth of understanding from psychology and organizational management on the individual and systemic features associated with increasing risk of error and harm, and there is thus relatively little to be gained from additional descriptive/qualitative work of this sort. The appropriate emphasis that has existed to date on systems change is ripe for review. There is no doubt that much of the impact of adverse events is inherent in the systems within which people work, and that there is a real and remaining need to move away from a blame culture that sees individuals as responsible for the impact of incidents. However, there is also a need to look at the interplay between the individual and systemic characteristics and what features are associated with safe practice and resilient organizations: for example, individuals often act as the major protective barrier to prevent error impacting upon patients through their interventions within the system or through their safety vigilance. How we can enhance or develop this role is worthy of investigation (Box 12.5).

Box 12.5 **Research priorities for patient safety**

- Understanding when adverse events occur
- Understanding what causes adverse events
- Developing methods of preventing adverse events
- Ensuring that change is sustained in both individuals and organizations

(After Walshe & Boaden, 2006.)

Box 12.6 **The need for clear goals for improvement in patient safety**

'The most important single step that should be taken by the United States to align the forces of change would be to set and adhere to strict, ambitious, quantitative, and well-tracked national goals.'
(From Leape & Berwick, 2005.)

The real priority for the coming decade is, however, demonstrating to government, policy-makers and the public alike that it is possible to translate these insights into interventions that can potentially and actually enhance patient safety. Here some progress has been achieved, but even in the arena of medicines management errors, which is one of the best-studied fields, there is very little high-quality evidence on how to reduce the burden posed by these errors. This reflects the difficulty of demonstrating the impact of complex interventions and the currently limited evidence base for the effectiveness of safety interventions. Because many interventions will by necessity be complex interventions they will need a combination of quantitative and qualitative approaches to allow meaningful study of the best ways of implementing the most promising interventions so as to enable long-term sustainability of change.

Conclusions

Although the study of patient safety has come a long way over the last two decades it remains a discipline in its infancy. The next decade of policy and research will be crucial to determining whether the insights thus far gained can be translated into initiatives that actually improve outcomes for patients, which will be essential to the long-term sustainability of the discipline. In many areas, the science is too underdeveloped to allow interventions to be rigorously evaluated, a point that must be recognized by potential funders, who will need to be convinced to invest for the long term (Box 12.6).

Conflict of interest

AS has none. RT and MB are employed by the National Patient Safety Agency, which is responsible for leading healthcare policy, data analysis and solution developments for safety.

Further reading

Department of Health. *An Organisation with a Memory*. Stationery Office, London, 2000.

Elwyn G, Corrigan MJ. The patient safety story. *Br Med J* 2005;**331**:302–304.

Institute of Medicine. *Patient Safety: Achieving a New Standard for Care*. National Academy Press, Washington DC, 2004.

Kohn LT, Corrigan JM, Donaldson MS (eds). *To Err is Human: Building a Safer Health System*. National Academies Press, Washington DC, 2000.

Leape LL, Berwick DM. Five years after *To Err Is Human*: what have we learned? *JAMA* 2005;**293**:2384–2390.

Rochlin GI. Safe operation as a social construct. *Ergonomics* 1999;**42**:1549–1560.

Walshe K, Boaden R (eds). *Patient Safety: Research into Practice*. Open University Press, Maidenhead, 2006.

Index

Note: page numbers in *italics* refer to figures, tables and boxes